BRAVE O.

Strength Training for Seniors Over 60

Adapted Programs for Older Adults with Limited Endurance

Contents

1

INTRODUCTION

Why Strength Training Matters After 60

Welcome to *Strength Training for Seniors over 60: Adapted Programs for Older Adults with Limited Endurance*. You've taken the first step toward a stronger, healthier, and more vibrant version of yourself, and that alone deserves a moment of celebration. Aging is a privilege, a testament to the life you've lived, the challenges you've overcome, and the wisdom you've gained. Yet, as the candles on our birthday cakes multiply, so do the whispers of change in our bodies. The muscles that once carried us effortlessly through life begin to lose their strength, joints may creak like an old staircase, and daily tasks that were once second nature can start to feel like mini challenges. But here's the truth—none of this has to define you.

Strength training after 60 isn't just about lifting weights or breaking a sweat; it's about reclaiming your vitality, preserving your independence, and refusing to let age dictate what you can and cannot do. It's about standing tall—both literally and figuratively—and saying, "I am still strong, and I will remain so."

Let's start with a myth that needs busting: getting older means slowing down. Absolutely not! The idea that fitness is reserved for the young is outdated nonsense. Research consistently shows that strength training is one of the most effective ways to combat the natural effects of aging. It builds muscle, strengthens bones, improves balance, and keeps your heart healthy. Most importantly, it enhances your quality of life. Imagine carrying groceries without a second thought, playing with your grandkids without running out of breath, or simply moving through your day with confidence and ease. Strength training makes all this possible—and more.

But let's be real for a moment. Starting—or restarting—a fitness journey at this stage in life can feel daunting. Perhaps you've had moments of doubt, thinking, "Is it safe for me to do this?" or "What if I injure myself?" These concerns are valid, and they stem from a place of care for your well-being. That's why this book exists—to guide you step by step, offering practical, safe, and effective programs designed specifically for older adults with limited endurance.

You don't need to be a gym rat or lift heavy weights to see remarkable benefits. Sometimes, small, consistent efforts are the most powerful. Simple exercises, like using resistance bands or even your own body weight, can yield incredible results when done correctly. You'll feel stronger, more agile, and more in control of your body, regardless of where you're starting from.

But here's the best part: strength training is more than a physical transformation. It's emotional and mental as well. Every time you complete a workout, you're not just building muscle—you're building confidence. You're proving to yourself that you are capable, resilient, and ready to face life's challenges head-on. That sense of empowerment ripples through every aspect of your life, reminding you that age is just a number, not a limitation.

As you embark on this journey, remember that progress is personal. It's not about comparing yourself to anyone else but about becoming the strongest, healthiest version of yourself. There will be days when it feels hard, and that's okay. On those days, remind yourself why you started. You're not just training for today—you're training for the years ahead. You're investing in your ability to live independently, pursue your passions, and embrace the joy of movement.

So, take a deep breath and pat yourself on the back for taking this first step. You've already shown incredible courage and commitment by opening this book and deciding to prioritize your health. Together, we'll explore adapted programs that meet you where you are, challenge you safely, and help you achieve results that matter.

Strength training after 60 isn't just an activity; it's a celebration of life. It's a testament to your determination to keep moving forward, stronger and more vibrant with each passing day.

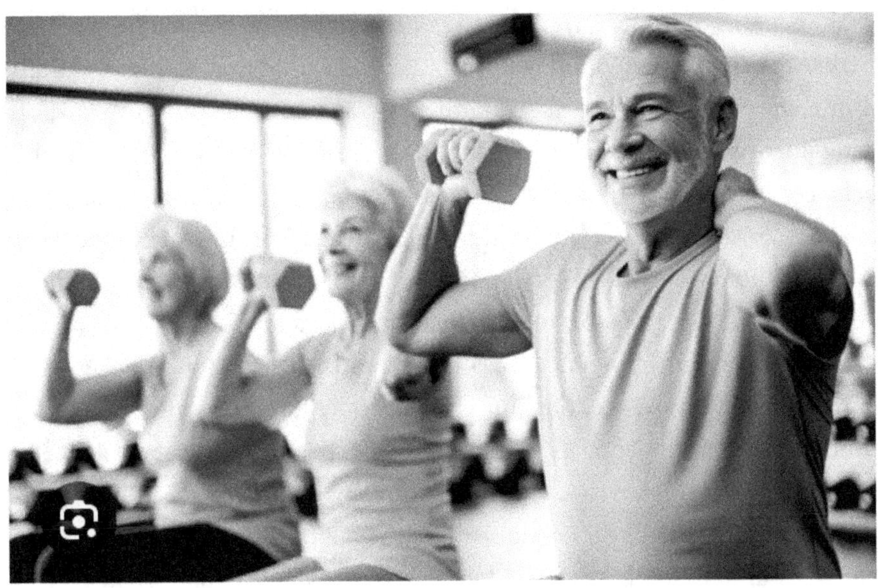

Understanding the Benefits of Strength Training

When you hear the words "strength training," you might picture a gym packed with bulky bodybuilders grunting under heavy barbells. Let's set the record straight—strength training isn't just for the young, the fit, or the iron-pumping elite. It's for everyone, especially those of us who have gathered the wisdom of 60 or more years. In fact, it's one of the most powerful tools we have to maintain independence, vitality, and joy in our golden years.

Here's the simple truth: your body is a marvel of resilience and adaptability. Even as we age, it retains an incredible ability to grow stronger and more capable, provided we give it the right care and attention. Strength training isn't just about building muscle; it's about building a life where your body works with you, not against you. It's about standing from a chair without hesitation, walking up stairs without holding your breath, and feeling a renewed sense of control over how you move and live.

The benefits of strength training after 60 go far beyond the obvious physical perks. Yes, it will help you maintain and even rebuild muscle that naturally diminishes with age. Yes, it strengthens your bones, helping to ward off osteoporosis and reducing the risk of fractures. And yes, it improves your balance, lowering the likelihood of falls—a concern that becomes more real as the years go by. But it's more than that. Strength training reshapes how you feel about yourself. Every time you complete a workout, you remind yourself that you're capable, determined, and vibrant.

Let's talk about the science for a moment, because it's fascinating—and empowering. As we age, our muscles naturally lose mass and strength, a process called sarcopenia. Left unchecked, this decline can make daily tasks more difficult and increase your risk of injury. But here's the good news: strength training is like a magic spell that reverses this process. When you engage your muscles through resistance exercises, you stimulate them to grow stronger, countering the effects of sarcopenia. It's not just about preserving what you have—it's about gaining back what you thought was gone.

Beyond the muscles, strength training works wonders for your bones. Did you know that your bones, like your muscles, respond to challenges? When you lift weights or perform resistance exercises, your bones adapt by becoming denser and stronger. This is crucial for maintaining your independence and avoiding fractures that can sideline even the most active senior. It's like giving your skeleton a shield of resilience to carry you through the years.

But perhaps one of the most underestimated benefits of strength training is its impact on your mind. Exercise has a remarkable ability to boost your mood, reduce anxiety, and sharpen your cognitive function. Strength training, in particular, gives you a sense of accomplishment and control, lifting your spirits and reminding you that age is just a number. Each session becomes a victory—a statement to yourself that you are not defined by limitations, but by your determination to keep moving forward.

Now, let's address the elephant in the room: endurance. If you're worried about not being able to keep up or feeling too tired to start, let me reassure you—this program is designed with you in mind. Strength training for seniors isn't about pushing past your limits; it's about working within them, gently expanding your capacity over time. You don't need to spend hours lifting heavy weights or sweating profusely. Simple, tailored exercises, done consistently, can deliver life-changing results.

Imagine this: waking up each morning feeling energized and confident in your ability to tackle the day. Imagine bending down to pick up something from the floor without worrying about your back. Imagine playing with your grandchildren or taking that long-awaited trip without second-guessing whether your body will cooperate. These aren't just dreams—they're achievable realities with the right approach to strength training.

This book isn't here to lecture or overwhelm you. It's here to guide you, step by step, through a journey that will transform not just your body but your entire perspective on aging. Strength training isn't about denying the passage of time—it's about embracing it with grace, power, and determination. It's about proving to yourself, and perhaps to others, that you still have so much more to give, so much more to experience, and so much more to enjoy.

Dispelling Myths About Fitness for Seniors

Let's get one thing straight: age is not a stop sign for fitness. Yet, so many myths about exercise and aging have wormed their way into our collective thinking, convincing older adults that staying active is either too dangerous, too pointless, or just plain impossible. It's time to put those myths to rest—

because not only is fitness achievable after 60, but it's also one of the most important things you can do for your health, happiness, and independence.

One of the biggest myths out there is that it's "too late" to start exercising. People say it all the time: "Oh, I'm past my prime," or "What's the point now?" Let me be blunt—that's nonsense. The human body is an incredible machine, designed to adapt and improve at any age. Whether you're 30, 60, or 90, your muscles, bones, and heart respond to movement. Studies have shown that even people in their 80s and 90s can gain strength and improve balance with regular exercise. So no, it's not too late. In fact, this might be the perfect time to start.

Another pervasive myth is that strength training is too risky for seniors. Maybe you've heard that lifting weights will strain your heart, damage your joints, or leave you hobbling around the next day. Let me tell you something: sitting on the couch all day is far riskier. Weak muscles and brittle bones are a recipe for falls, fractures, and losing the independence you've worked so hard to maintain. Strength training, when done correctly and safely, is one of the best ways to protect your body and keep it functioning beautifully. With the right guidance—like the programs in this book—you can build strength without fear.

And then there's the classic excuse: "I'm too old to see results." Really? Because science says otherwise. You might not be training to set world records or compete in bodybuilding competitions (unless you want to!), but strength training offers real, measurable benefits for seniors. From improving balance and reducing fall risks to increasing muscle mass and even sharpening your mind, the results are undeniable. You'll move better, feel better, and— let's be honest—look better, too. That's not vanity; that's confidence, and you deserve to feel great about yourself at any age.

Of course, we can't ignore the myth that fitness has to be grueling to work. Somewhere along the line, people got the idea that exercise has to hurt to be effective. No pain, no gain, right? Wrong. The truth is, effective strength training for seniors is about smart, tailored exercises that meet you where you are. It's not about lifting the heaviest weights or doing endless reps—it's about building strength gradually, listening to your body, and focusing on consistent progress. You don't need to spend hours in a gym or push through unbearable discomfort. This isn't boot camp; it's a celebration of what your body can do.

Let's not forget the more subtle myth: that fitness is only about the body. Yes, strength training improves physical health, but its benefits extend far beyond your muscles and bones. Regular exercise boosts mood, reduces anxiety, and sharpens memory. It helps you sleep better and face each day with more energy. When you challenge your body, you empower your mind. Every step, stretch, or lift is a declaration: "I'm not done yet." It's a reminder that your best days are still ahead of you, not behind.

You may have encountered skepticism from others—or even from yourself—about whether fitness is worth the effort at this stage of life. It is. Fitness isn't about trying to turn back the clock; it's about embracing the future with strength, grace, and confidence. Forget what society says about aging. You're not fragile, you're not too old, and you're certainly not out of options. You're a powerhouse in the making, and this journey is about unlocking that potential.

So, let's dispel these myths together. Fitness after 60 isn't a fairy tale; it's a fact backed by science, success stories, and the innate resilience of the human spirit. You don't need a perfect body or boundless energy to get started. All you need is a willingness to try—and that, my friend, is where the magic begins.

By the time you finish this book, those myths will be a distant memory, replaced by a sense of empowerment and a newfound belief in what you're capable of. Because here's the truth: the best time to invest in your strength, health, and happiness is now. Let's get to work—myths be damned!

How to Use This Book

This book is your guide, your coach, and your companion on a journey designed specifically for you. Whether you've been active your whole life or are just starting to explore fitness, this book meets you where you are and helps you move forward with confidence.

But let's address the elephant in the room: fitness books can be overwhelming. You may have flipped through a few in the past only to be bombarded with jargon, intimidating workout plans, and unrealistic expectations. That's not what you'll find here. This isn't about forcing you into a cookie-cutter program or throwing you into the deep end of fitness trends. This book is about understanding *you*—your unique needs, abilities, and goals—and creating a roadmap that works for your body and your life.

Think of this book as a friendly coach sitting beside you, not a drill sergeant barking orders. Every chapter has been carefully crafted to guide you through the "why," the "what," and the "how" of strength training. You'll learn why each exercise matters, how to perform it safely, and what benefits you can expect to see over time. If you've ever worried about injuring yourself or felt unsure about whether you're doing things correctly, those worries end here.

To get the most out of this book, take your time. This isn't a race, and there's no finish line you're required to cross by a certain date. Some days, you may feel energized and ready to dive into a full workout. Other days, you might prefer to revisit the foundational concepts or focus on stretching and recovery. Both are equally important. The beauty of this book is its flexibility—it adapts to your pace and grows with you.

As you move through the chapters, you'll notice that everything builds on a foundation of safety, simplicity, and gradual progress. This isn't about pushing your body to its limits or chasing extreme results. It's about developing sustainable habits that make you feel stronger and more capable every day. Along the way, you'll find practical tips for modifying exercises, staying motivated, and overcoming common challenges. These tools are here to make your journey enjoyable, not burdensome.

One thing to keep in mind is that progress looks different for everyone. Maybe you'll notice improvements in your balance and posture after just a few weeks. Maybe you'll feel a boost in your energy levels or find yourself moving through daily tasks with greater ease. Or maybe you'll start to feel an intangible but deeply satisfying sense of accomplishment—a reminder that you're investing in your health and future. Whatever progress looks like for you, celebrate it. Every step forward is a victory.

This book is more than just a collection of exercises and programs. It's a testament to the belief that age is not a barrier to strength and vitality. It's a reminder that you are capable of remarkable things, even if you've doubted yourself in the past. So, if you're feeling a mix of excitement and nervousness, know that you're not alone. That's exactly how most journeys worth taking begin.

As you work through the pages, allow yourself to experiment, to learn, and to grow. There's no "right" way to use this book—only the way that feels right for you. Whether you choose to read it cover to cover or jump straight to the exercises, this book is here to support you every step of the way.

So, grab your water bottle, find a comfortable spot, and take a deep breath. You've got this. Let's turn the page and begin a journey that's not just about fitness—it's about living your best, strongest, and happiest life. Together, we'll prove that strength doesn't fade with age; it evolves. And so can you.

2

Chapter 1: The Science of Aging and Strength

What Happens to Muscles as We Age

Aging is a natural process, but its effects on our muscles often catch us by surprise. One of the most significant changes is something called sarcopenia—the gradual loss of muscle mass and strength that begins as early as our 30s and accelerates after 60. While this may sound discouraging, understanding what's happening to your body is the first step toward addressing it. Sarcopenia isn't a death sentence for your strength; it's a call to action. With the right approach, you can counter its effects and even regain muscle you thought was gone for good.

Sarcopenia and its impact on strength.

Sarcopenia is the term used to describe the natural loss of muscle mass and strength that occurs as we age. While it's a normal part of the aging process, its impact can feel anything but normal when it starts to interfere with everyday life. This gradual decline in muscle tissue doesn't just affect your ability to lift heavy objects—it affects your ability to maintain balance, perform simple tasks, and live independently. Sarcopenia can turn what once felt easy—getting out of a chair, climbing stairs, or carrying groceries—into a real challenge.

The process of sarcopenia often begins as early as your 30s, with muscle mass declining at a slow but steady rate. By the time you reach your 60s and beyond, the rate of muscle loss accelerates significantly if no action is taken. What's important to understand is that this isn't just about losing muscle size—it's about losing muscle function. As muscles weaken, so does their ability to generate force, which directly impacts your strength. This loss doesn't just happen in your arms or legs; it affects the core muscles that stabilize your body and the small muscles that keep your movements coordinated and precise.

The consequences of sarcopenia extend beyond the inconvenience of reduced strength. Weak muscles increase your risk of falls and injuries, which can lead to a downward spiral of reduced mobility and independence. For many seniors, this cascade of events marks the difference between aging actively and aging with significant physical limitations. Sarcopenia also contributes to slower metabolism, making it easier to gain unwanted fat and harder to maintain overall health.

The good news is that sarcopenia isn't irreversible. Muscle tissue is highly adaptable, even in older adults. Strength training has been proven to combat sarcopenia effectively by stimulating muscle growth and improving function. Regular resistance exercises can help rebuild lost muscle and restore strength, allowing you to reclaim mobility, confidence, and quality of life. The key is starting where you are, focusing on proper form and consistency, and combining your efforts with good nutrition to support muscle repair and growth.

Sarcopenia doesn't have to define your later years. With the right mindset and approach, you can push back against its effects and regain the strength to live life on your terms.

How inactivity accelerates muscle loss.

Inactivity is one of the primary drivers of accelerated muscle loss as we age, and it's a challenge that many seniors face, often unknowingly. The human body is incredibly adaptable, which means if we don't use our muscles, they start to weaken and deteriorate faster than if we were active. Think of your muscles as a skill or a tool: if you don't practice or use them regularly, they'll lose their sharpness and effectiveness. Unfortunately, inactivity becomes a vicious cycle—weak muscles make it harder to stay active, and less activity leads to even weaker muscles.

When you stop moving, your muscles begin to atrophy—this means they actually shrink in size. This shrinkage isn't just a cosmetic issue; it reflects a loss of muscle fibers and a reduction in muscle strength. The decline isn't immediate but gradually creeps in as days turn into weeks and weeks turn into months of physical inactivity. Even if you're not bedridden, spending extended periods sitting—whether that's in front of the TV, at a desk, or in a car—still has a profound impact on muscle health. Prolonged periods of inactivity slow down blood flow, reduce oxygen supply to muscles, and impair nutrient delivery, which all contribute to muscle deterioration.

As muscles weaken, they lose their ability to generate force, which affects everything from lifting grocery bags to simply getting up from a chair. Without regular use, muscle fibers become less responsive to exercise signals, and muscle protein synthesis—the process of building and repairing muscle tissue—slows down. This can lead to a noticeable drop in muscle tone and overall strength. The problem is compounded by age, as older adults naturally become less physically active due to changes in metabolism, joint stiffness, and energy levels.

To make matters worse, inactivity doesn't just impact muscles—it affects bones as well. Our bones and muscles work together; strong muscles support bone density, which can also decline with inactivity. When muscles weaken, they can no longer protect bones as effectively, increasing the risk of fractures and falls. The combination of muscle and bone loss makes movement more precarious and daily activities more challenging, creating a cycle that's difficult to break.

The good news is that strength training is a powerful antidote to the dangers of inactivity. Even small, gradual increases in physical activity can stimulate muscle growth, improve strength, and reverse the effects of sarcopenia. By reintroducing movement and resistance exercises into your routine, you can halt muscle atrophy, boost circulation, and maintain a healthy metabolic rate. It's about breaking the cycle of inactivity and taking proactive steps to protect your muscles and bones for the long haul.

The role of nutrition in muscle maintenance.

Nutrition plays a crucial role in muscle maintenance, especially as we age. Your body needs more than just exercise to keep muscles healthy and functioning optimally—it also requires the right balance of nutrients to support muscle growth, repair, and maintenance. This is because, as we age, our bodies become less efficient at using the nutrients we consume, making proper nutrition even more important. Think of it as fueling a high-performance car; if you put the wrong fuel in the tank, the engine simply can't perform at its best. Similarly, if you don't provide the right nutrients to your muscles, they won't be able to grow or recover as effectively.

Protein is at the heart of muscle maintenance. It's the building block of muscle tissue, essential for repair and growth. When you engage in strength training, your muscle fibers experience tiny tears, and they need protein to rebuild stronger than before. Without adequate protein, this repair process slows down, and muscle loss accelerates. The recommended daily amount of protein increases with age, particularly for seniors, who may need up to 1.2 to 2.0 grams of protein per kilogram of body weight to maintain muscle mass. This may seem like a lot, but it's achievable with thoughtful meal planning and incorporating protein-rich foods into your diet.

But protein alone isn't enough. Your body also needs an array of other nutrients to keep muscles in top shape. Vitamins and minerals, such as vitamin D, calcium, and magnesium, are crucial for bone health and muscle function. Vitamin D, in particular, supports muscle function and immune health, which is vital for older adults who may not get enough sunlight exposure. Magnesium helps relax muscles after exercise, reducing the risk of cramps and stiffness. Calcium, on the other hand, is essential for muscle contraction and bone health, working in tandem with protein to ensure your muscles stay strong.

Furthermore, hydration is often overlooked but is essential for muscle maintenance. Water plays a key role in muscle function, helping with nutrient delivery, waste removal, and overall muscle contraction. Dehydration can lead to muscle cramps, weakness, and decreased physical performance. The goal is to drink enough water throughout the day, not just during or after exercise, to support optimal muscle health.

Finally, antioxidants play a role in muscle maintenance by protecting muscle cells from oxidative stress—a common issue as we age. Free radicals can damage muscle cells and accelerate muscle aging, so consuming foods rich in antioxidants, like fruits, vegetables, nuts, and seeds, can help mitigate this risk.

In summary, nutrition is the missing link in the muscle maintenance equation for seniors. Proper nutrition ensures that your body has the resources it needs to rebuild muscle tissue after workouts, support bone density, and keep you active and independent for years to come. By paying attention to your diet and making smart food choices, you can enhance your strength training efforts and maintain muscle mass throughout your later years.

Strength Training and Aging

Strength training is not just about lifting weights—it's about reversing the muscle decline that so often accompanies aging. As we get older, it's natural for our muscles to weaken and lose mass, but resistance training provides a powerful counterforce. By engaging in strength exercises, you stimulate muscle fibers to grow and strengthen, a process known as muscle hypertrophy. This doesn't just help maintain muscle mass—it can actually reverse some of the effects of sarcopenia, the age-related loss of muscle tissue. Through consistent resistance training, you can regain strength, improve muscle tone, and even increase your overall muscle size, helping you stay active and independent longer.

How resistance training reverses muscle decline.

Resistance training is a game-changer when it comes to reversing muscle decline associated with aging. Unlike other forms of exercise that primarily maintain muscle mass, resistance training actively stimulates muscle growth. This means that through lifting weights, using resistance bands, or even bodyweight exercises like squats and push-ups, you can build new muscle fibers or strengthen the existing ones. The key lies in the concept of muscle hypertrophy—your muscles are forced to adapt to the stress placed on them, which prompts them to grow in size and strength.

As you lift weights, you create small tears in muscle fibers. These fibers then repair themselves stronger than before, a process that increases muscle mass and strength over time. This repair and growth mechanism is especially effective in older adults, as it counteracts the natural atrophy that occurs with inactivity or aging. It's not just about maintaining the muscle you have; resistance training allows you to build new muscle, reversing the effects of sarcopenia and reclaiming strength that may have been lost over the years. This process can make it easier to perform daily activities, enhance physical function, and improve overall quality of life.

In addition to muscle mass, resistance training has a profound impact on muscle function. It strengthens muscles by increasing their capacity to generate force, which is essential for maintaining balance, stability, and coordination. This is particularly important as we age because it helps prevent falls and injuries—two common issues that seniors face due to muscle weakness. Stronger muscles also take pressure off joints, which can reduce pain and improve mobility. By reversing muscle decline, you enhance not just your physical appearance but also your ability to move freely and enjoy life without limitations.

Furthermore, resistance training can even have a neurological impact. It stimulates the nervous system, which sends signals to muscles, making them more responsive and less prone to weakness. This can improve reaction times and reduce the risk of accidents. By keeping the nervous system active, you're not just improving muscle health but also enhancing overall functional capacity. Resistance training isn't a miracle cure, but it is a powerful tool for reversing muscle decline, keeping you strong, agile, and independent as you age. It's about taking charge of your health and not letting the years dictate your level of fitness.

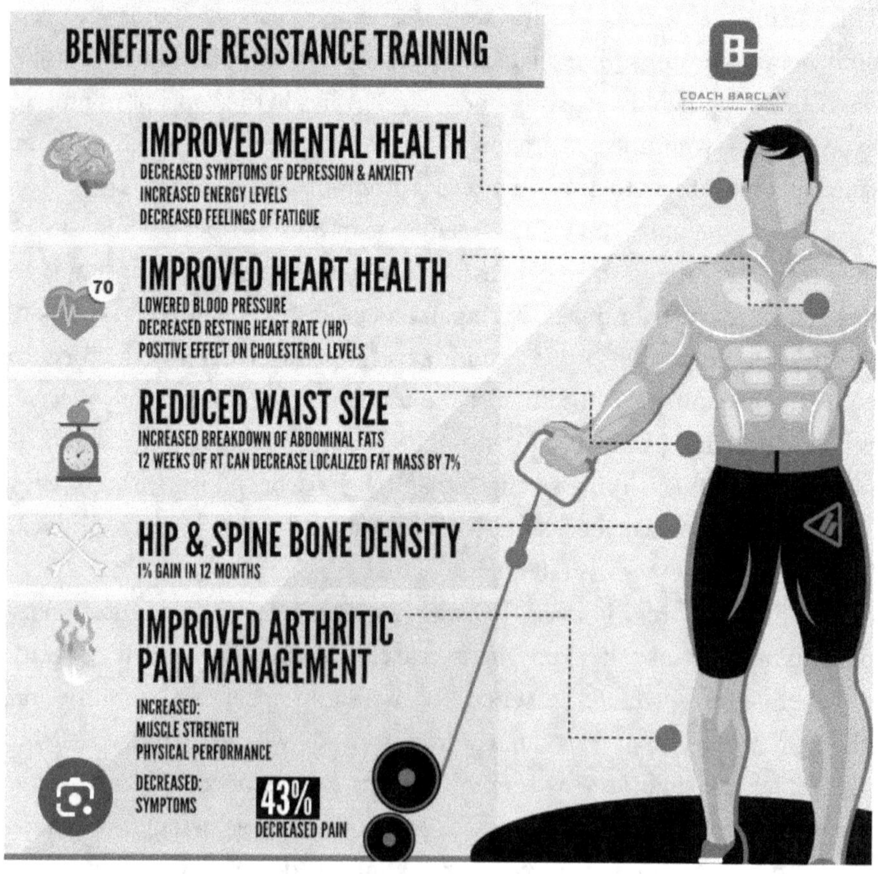

The impact on bone density and joint health.

Strength training has a significant positive impact on bone density and joint health, two key areas that often decline with age. When you engage in resistance exercises, such as lifting weights or using resistance bands, you create mechanical stress on bones. This stress stimulates a process known as bone remodeling, where old bone tissue is broken down and new, stronger bone is formed in its place. This is crucial for maintaining bone density and reducing the risk of osteoporosis, a condition characterized by weakened bones and increased fracture risk.

As we age, bone density naturally decreases due to hormonal changes and reduced physical activity. This makes bones more susceptible to fractures, especially if there's a fall. Strength training helps counteract this by increasing bone mineral density, particularly in the hips, spine, and wrists, which are common fracture sites for seniors. The more weight-bearing exercises you do, the more your bones adapt, becoming denser and stronger. This is not only about reducing the risk of fractures but also about maintaining a stable structure that supports your muscles, joints, and overall mobility.

Joint health is also a key beneficiary of strength training. As we age, joints can become stiff and less flexible, making simple activities challenging. Resistance exercises increase the synovial fluid around joints, which acts as a natural lubricant, keeping them flexible and reducing pain and stiffness. Strong muscles also protect joints from excessive wear and tear, providing stability and support. By reinforcing the muscles around the joints, you alleviate pressure and stress on them, helping to prevent injuries and maintain better joint function.

In addition to bone density and joint health, strength training supports overall skeletal health. It helps maintain proper posture and alignment, reducing the risk of conditions like osteoporosis and scoliosis. By engaging in a regular strength training routine, you're not just building muscle but also reinforcing the entire musculoskeletal system, ensuring that bones, muscles, and joints work together harmoniously. This holistic approach to fitness is key to aging well and maintaining an active, independent lifestyle.

Benefits for cardiovascular health and energy levels.

Strength training offers significant benefits for cardiovascular health and energy levels, areas that are critical for overall well-being as we age. While it's commonly associated with muscle building, resistance training also plays a key role in improving heart health and boosting energy levels, making it an essential part of a senior's fitness routine.

Engaging in strength training exercises increases your heart rate, which promotes better circulation and improves cardiovascular efficiency. This means that as your heart works harder to pump blood, it becomes stronger and more capable of delivering oxygen and nutrients to your muscles and organs. Over time, this can lead to lower resting heart rates, reduced blood pressure, and improved cholesterol levels—all of which contribute to a healthier heart. By reducing strain on the cardiovascular system, strength training lowers the risk of heart disease, stroke, and other related conditions, ensuring that your heart remains strong and efficient well into your later years.

In addition to heart health, strength training has a direct impact on energy levels. As you build muscle, your body becomes more efficient at burning calories, even at rest. This means that you can enjoy more energy throughout the day without feeling fatigued. Muscle tissue is metabolically active, so the more muscle mass you have, the more calories your body burns, helping you maintain a healthy weight. This increased caloric expenditure not only supports weight management but also enhances your overall vitality and sense of well-being. You'll find that daily activities become easier, energy levels remain steadier, and you're less prone to feelings of fatigue and lethargy.

Moreover, strength training helps stabilize blood sugar levels and improve insulin sensitivity, which is particularly important for older adults who are at a higher risk of developing type 2 diabetes. Regular exercise, including strength training, helps manage blood sugar spikes and improves the body's ability to use insulin effectively, reducing the risk of diabetes and its associated complications. It's not just about looking good or maintaining strength; strength training is a powerful tool for managing chronic conditions and promoting overall health.

By integrating strength training into your fitness routine, you're setting yourself up for better cardiovascular health and enhanced energy levels. The benefits extend beyond mere muscle building to include improved heart health, better circulation, and a steady supply of energy for daily activities. This means more active days, more stamina for social engagements, and a higher quality of life as you age. Strength training isn't just about aesthetics; it's about optimizing your physical health and making the most of every day.

CARDIOVASCULAR BENEFITS OF EXERCISE

HEART	BLOOD VESSELS	BLOOD
↑ Cardiac output ↑ Cardiac contraction/relaxation velocity ↑ Organ perfusion ↑ Cardiac growth and size ↓ Resting heart rate	↑ Vessel wall relaxation & dilatation ↓ Vascular resistance ↓ Blood pressure ↓ Arteriosclerosis plaque formation and instability	↑ Insulin sensitivity ↑ Insulin dependent glucose uptake ↑ Glucose control ↑ Oxygen carrying capacity ↑ HDL ↓ LDL ↓ Triglyceride

Collectively reduce

Burden & risk factors for cardiovascular diseases

Improved Heart Health and Reduced Cardiovascular Related Deaths

Fitness Assessment for Seniors

Assessing your current fitness level as a senior is the first step towards developing a safe and effective strength training program. It's important to begin with an honest evaluation of where you stand physically so that you can make informed decisions about your fitness goals. This process involves understanding your strengths and limitations, which can vary widely from person to person. By starting with a fitness assessment, you gain a clear picture of what you can safely achieve, where you need to focus your efforts, and how to structure your exercises to align with your individual capabilities. This helps in tailoring a program that's right for you, one that respects any existing health conditions or mobility challenges you might have.

Assessing your current fitness level safely.

Assessing your current fitness level safely as a senior involves a thoughtful and measured approach that takes into account your health status, mobility, and any pre-existing conditions. The goal is to gather information that helps you understand where you stand physically so you can build an appropriate strength training program. It's about evaluating your strengths and weaknesses without pushing too hard or too fast, which could lead to injury or setbacks. The first step is to consult with a healthcare professional, such as a doctor or physical therapist, who can provide guidance based on your medical history and any conditions that might impact your ability to exercise. This professional input ensures that your assessment is not only safe but also tailored to your specific needs.

Start by performing a basic self-assessment to gauge your current level of physical activity. This might include simple tasks like walking around your home, climbing a few stairs, or doing a few sit-to-stand exercises. These tasks give you an idea of your endurance, balance, and strength. You can also track your heart rate and blood pressure to get an understanding of how your body responds to physical activity. This initial evaluation provides a benchmark that allows you to monitor your progress over time. It's important to note that even small movements can give you valuable insight into how your body reacts to exercise and where you may need to focus more effort.

Next, consider any physical limitations you might have. This could be joint stiffness, decreased range of motion, or a history of injury. Understanding these limitations helps you choose exercises that are safe and effective without exacerbating any existing conditions. Avoid exercises that put excessive strain on joints or muscles, especially if you have arthritis or past injuries. The goal is to build strength gradually and in a way that supports long-term health and mobility. Once you've identified your limitations, you can select exercises that align with your abilities, like low-impact cardio or bodyweight exercises, to build a foundation before progressing to more challenging activities.

Finally, it's essential to recognize that assessing your fitness level safely is an ongoing process. Regularly checking in with yourself and adjusting your routine as needed is key to preventing overexertion and maintaining steady progress. As you get stronger, you may need to modify exercises to continue challenging your body without risking injury. This might involve increasing weights, changing the type of exercises, or varying the intensity. By taking a cautious and adaptable approach, you can create a sustainable exercise routine that supports your long-term fitness goals and helps you maintain independence and quality of life as you age.

Recognizing limitations and avoiding overexertion.

Recognizing limitations and avoiding overexertion is a crucial aspect of designing a safe and effective fitness routine for seniors. As we age, our bodies become more susceptible to injury, and our physical capabilities change. It's important to be realistic about what we can and can't do without risking harm. This means taking stock of any health issues, mobility restrictions, or past injuries that might impact how we approach exercise. The first step is to acknowledge these limitations without feeling defeated; they are part of your unique fitness journey and should guide your choices in exercises and routines.

To recognize limitations, start by listening to your body. Pain, discomfort, or fatigue that lingers after an activity are signs that you may have pushed too hard. It's important to differentiate between the normal muscle burn from an effective workout and pain that could be indicative of an injury or strain. This means paying attention to how you feel during and after exercise. If certain movements or exercises cause pain or exacerbate existing conditions like arthritis, joint stiffness, or osteoporosis, it's essential to modify or avoid them. There's no shame in opting for easier versions of exercises or consulting with a fitness professional to find suitable alternatives.

Avoiding overexertion goes hand in hand with recognizing limitations. Pushing too hard, especially when you're just starting a new exercise routine, can lead to injuries such as strains, sprains, or worse—muscle tears. Overexertion can also contribute to burnout, which might make you less likely to stick to your fitness goals in the long run. The key is to start slow and gradually increase the intensity, duration, and frequency of your workouts. This gradual approach allows your body to adapt, recover, and build strength safely. It's about challenging yourself in a way that doesn't compromise your health or well-being. Listen to your body's signals and respect them; they're your best guide to avoiding overexertion and making sustainable progress.

Ultimately, recognizing limitations and avoiding overexertion is about taking a balanced approach to exercise. It's about finding the sweet spot between challenging yourself and protecting your body from potential harm. By being mindful of your physical boundaries and adjusting your workout routine accordingly, you can enjoy the benefits of strength training—like increased muscle strength, better bone density, and improved cardiovascular health—without risking injury. It's a process that requires patience, but the rewards are worth it. The goal is not just to exercise but to do so in a way that supports your health and allows you to live an active, vibrant life well into your senior years.

Setting personalized, achievable fitness benchmarks.

Setting personalized, achievable fitness benchmarks is a fundamental part of any successful strength training program for seniors. It's about creating realistic goals that are tailored to your individual needs, capabilities, and aspirations. The first step in this process is to understand what you want to achieve with your fitness routine. Whether it's regaining mobility, increasing endurance, losing weight, or simply feeling stronger and more energetic, your benchmarks should align with these specific objectives. This approach ensures that you're not just exercising for the sake of it but are working towards measurable outcomes that matter to you personally.

To set effective benchmarks, start with an honest assessment of where you currently stand. This involves evaluating your current physical condition, including your strength, flexibility, balance, and cardiovascular health. It's important to be realistic about your starting point; don't set goals that are too ambitious without a solid plan to achieve them. For example, if you're just beginning strength training, aiming to lift heavy weights from the start might not be achievable or safe. Instead, set initial goals that focus on form and technique, gradually progressing to heavier weights or more challenging exercises as your strength and confidence improve. The idea is to build a foundation that you can build upon steadily over time.

Next, break down your long-term goals into smaller, more manageable milestones. These should be specific, measurable, achievable, relevant, and time-bound—often referred to as SMART goals. For instance, if your long-term goal is to improve overall strength, a SMART benchmark might be to lift a certain weight for a specified number of repetitions by a certain date. Short-term goals can include things like completing a certain number of sets or reps without discomfort, walking a certain distance, or doing a specific exercise without modifications. These milestones provide a clear sense of direction and allow you to track progress over time. They also help keep you motivated by giving you something tangible to aim for and celebrate as you meet each goal.

Finally, as you set these benchmarks, remember that they should be adaptable. Life happens, and sometimes things don't go as planned. Be open to adjusting your goals if necessary. If an exercise is too challenging or if you experience discomfort, modify the goal or try a different approach. The flexibility to adjust benchmarks as you progress is key to maintaining a sustainable and effective strength training routine. By continually assessing and tweaking your benchmarks, you ensure that you're working within a framework that supports long-term health and wellness. The ultimate goal is to make progress at your own pace, safely and sustainably, while staying motivated and enjoying the benefits of strength training.

3

Chapter 2: Preparing Your Body and Mind for Strength Training

Safety First: Precautions for Senior Fitness

When it comes to senior fitness, safety should always come first. Before you start any new exercise program, it's crucial to consult with your doctor, especially if you have underlying health conditions or haven't been active for a while. Your doctor can provide personalized advice based on your medical history and current health status. They can help you understand any limitations you might have and recommend exercises that are safe and effective for your individual needs. This consultation is not just a formality; it's an essential step in ensuring that your fitness routine supports your health without putting you at risk. Your doctor's guidance can help you navigate any potential pitfalls and set you up for a successful and injury-free exercise journey.

Consulting with your doctor before starting.

Consulting with your doctor before starting any fitness program is a vital precaution for seniors. This step is more than just a safety measure—it's an investment in your long-term health. Your doctor can provide personalized guidance based on your medical history, current health status, and any pre-existing conditions that could impact your ability to exercise. It's important to approach this conversation with honesty and openness about your lifestyle, physical activity level, and any concerns you may have. Your doctor will consider factors like chronic conditions, medications, and past injuries to ensure that your exercise routine is safe and effective for your specific needs.

During this consultation, your doctor can help identify any potential risks associated with physical activity. For instance, if you have a history of heart disease, high blood pressure, diabetes, osteoporosis, or arthritis, your doctor can recommend modifications to exercises or suggest alternative forms of physical activity that are gentler on your joints and cardiovascular system. They might also provide tips on how to manage medication schedules to avoid complications during exercise. This personalized advice helps you avoid overexertion and ensures that your workouts support your health rather than compromising it.

Additionally, consulting with your doctor can provide reassurance and guidance on what to watch for during exercise. They can explain warning signs that could indicate issues such as dehydration, heat intolerance, or an adverse reaction to exercise. By establishing clear guidelines, your doctor helps you make informed decisions about when to push yourself and when to take it easy. This advice sets the stage for a balanced fitness routine that aligns with your medical needs and physical abilities. Ultimately, consulting with your doctor is a proactive step that not only minimizes the risk of injury but also sets you up for a sustainable and enjoyable fitness journey.

Recognizing warning signs during exercise.

Recognizing warning signs during exercise is crucial for seniors to maintain their safety and health. These signs act as your body's way of communicating that something may be wrong. It's important to pay close attention to how you feel during physical activity to avoid potential complications. One of the primary warning signs is persistent pain—whether it's sharp, dull, or achy. Muscle discomfort that doesn't subside after a few minutes of rest or worsens during exercise could indicate overexertion, an injury, or an underlying health issue that needs immediate attention. Don't ignore these signals; your body is trying to protect itself from strain or damage.

Shortness of breath is another red flag that something may be wrong. While a moderate level of breathlessness can be expected with physical activity, sudden and severe difficulty in breathing or a sensation of suffocation could be a sign of cardiovascular distress or an acute respiratory issue. If you find yourself gasping for air, take a break immediately, sit down, and try to relax. If symptoms don't improve quickly, seek medical help. Additionally, dizziness or lightheadedness is concerning, especially if it happens without any known cause. It could indicate issues such as dehydration, low blood pressure, or an adverse reaction to the exercise. Never push through dizziness; it's a clear indication that your body is struggling.

Another important warning sign to watch for is chest pain or discomfort. This is particularly significant and should not be ignored. Chest pain could be a sign of heart strain or angina, and it's not something to take lightly. If you experience pressure, tightness, or a sharp pain in your chest during exercise, it's crucial to stop immediately, rest, and seek medical attention as soon as possible. Feeling unusually fatigued, especially if it's out of proportion to the effort being exerted, can also be a warning. This might be your body's way of signaling that it's not coping well with the workout and needs a break. Recognizing these warning signs allows you to take action quickly, preventing further injury and ensuring that you maintain a safe and effective exercise routine. Always prioritize your health and don't hesitate to consult a healthcare professional if you're in doubt.

Building a safe workout environment.

Building a safe workout environment is essential to prevent accidents and injuries during exercise, especially for seniors who may have reduced mobility or balance issues. The first step is to assess your workout space. It should be well-lit, free from obstacles, and have enough room for you to move around without risk of tripping or bumping into things. Clear away any clutter, like cords, toys, or furniture, that could cause trips or falls. This also includes securing rugs or carpets that may slip easily, as they can be a hazard when doing exercises that require you to step, jump, or squat. A clean and organized space not only reduces the risk of injury but also allows you to focus on your exercises without distractions.

Next, consider the flooring. Opt for a non-slip surface that provides good traction. Hardwood, tile, or vinyl floors can be slippery, so you might want to place an exercise mat over them to reduce the risk of slipping and provide some cushioning for joint protection. Rubber or foam mats can also absorb shock and reduce impact during exercises like squats or lunges. If you exercise outside, ensure that the area is smooth and free from hazards such as cracks, pebbles, or uneven terrain that could lead to falls. Safety is not just about preventing injuries; it's also about making sure that your workout space is inviting and comfortable for you to move around in safely.

Building a safe workout environment also means having the right equipment on hand. This includes using supportive gear like stability balls, resistance bands, dumbbells, or weights that are appropriate for your strength level. If you're new to exercise, consider using lighter weights or opting for resistance bands, which offer a safer, more controlled way to build strength without heavy lifting. Having a sturdy chair or handrails nearby can provide support and balance, especially if you need it for exercises like leg lifts or seated squats. Additionally, having a water bottle close by is important to stay hydrated throughout your workout, which can prevent dizziness and fatigue. A well-prepared environment ensures that you can exercise safely and comfortably, minimizing the risk of injury and making the most of your fitness routine.

Developing a Positive Mindset

Developing a positive mindset is key when it comes to embarking on a fitness journey, especially for seniors who might feel hesitant or doubtful about starting a new exercise program. It's natural to have concerns—whether it's fear of injury, worry about not being able to keep up, or just the uncertainty of trying something new. The first step in overcoming these fears is to acknowledge them and face them head-on. Recognize that starting small and progressing gradually is a completely valid approach. Remind yourself that everyone starts somewhere, and it's perfectly okay to take baby steps. The goal is not perfection from day one but steady progress and improvement over time.

Overcoming fear or doubt about starting fitness programs.

Overcoming fear or doubt about starting a fitness program is a common challenge, especially for seniors who may have had negative experiences with exercise in the past or who are simply unsure about their ability to begin a new routine. It's important to recognize that these feelings are natural and to approach them with patience and self-compassion. The first step in overcoming fear is to acknowledge it. Allow yourself to feel the anxiety or uncertainty without judgment. Understanding that these feelings are normal can be reassuring and provides an opportunity to address them head-on. Fear often stems from uncertainty about the unknown—worrying about potential discomfort, injury, or failure. By acknowledging these concerns, you can start to address them more effectively.

A key strategy in overcoming fear is to break down the barriers to entry. Start with small, manageable steps that gradually introduce you to physical activity. This might mean beginning with gentle stretches, seated exercises, or even just a short walk around the block. The goal is to build familiarity and comfort with movement at your own pace. By starting small, you allow yourself the time and space to adjust, both physically and mentally. As you build confidence through small successes, you can gradually increase the intensity and duration of your workouts. This incremental approach can make exercise feel less intimidating and more achievable.

Another powerful way to overcome doubt is to focus on the benefits rather than the challenges. Remind yourself of why you want to start this fitness journey in the first place—whether it's to improve your health, regain mobility, reduce pain, or simply feel more energetic. Reframing your mindset from what could go wrong to what could go right can significantly boost your motivation. Surround yourself with positive influences—whether it's a supportive fitness community, encouraging family members, or even a coach who can provide guidance and feedback. Their positive energy and belief in your ability to succeed can be contagious and help you push through moments of doubt. Ultimately, overcoming fear and doubt is about building trust in yourself and the process. It's about recognizing that you have the power to take control of your health and well-being, one step at a time.

Setting intentions and tracking progress.

Setting intentions and tracking progress are critical components of a successful fitness journey for seniors. These practices not only provide direction but also offer a means to stay motivated and accountable. Setting intentions is about clearly defining your goals and why they matter to you. It's about visualizing what you want to achieve and making a commitment to that outcome. Whether it's aiming to walk a certain distance each day, increase the number of repetitions for a particular exercise, or simply feel more energetic throughout the day, setting specific, measurable, and realistic goals gives you something concrete to strive for. This process helps you focus on what's most important and aligns your actions with your desired outcomes. It's about creating a personal roadmap that guides your efforts and keeps you on track.

Tracking progress is the other half of the equation. It's about monitoring your achievements and identifying areas for improvement. Keeping a log, journal, or using a fitness app can be incredibly helpful. Record the exercises you do, the amount of time you spend, the distances you cover, or the weights you lift. Track how you're feeling physically and emotionally. This can include anything from noticing how much easier it is to climb stairs to feeling less fatigued during the day. By documenting these milestones, you create a tangible record of your progress, which can be incredibly motivating. Seeing the numbers improve over time can be a powerful reminder of how far you've come, reinforcing the belief that your efforts are paying off.

Tracking progress also allows you to make adjustments when necessary. If you're not seeing the results you want, it's an opportunity to evaluate your routine and tweak it. Maybe you need to change the intensity, vary the exercises, or spend more time on certain activities. Regularly reviewing your progress gives you the chance to fine-tune your approach and adapt to what works best for you. It also allows you to celebrate your successes along the way. Every small win, whether it's lifting a little more weight, completing an extra lap, or simply feeling more confident, is a step toward achieving your larger fitness goals. By setting intentions and tracking progress, you create a clear sense of purpose and direction, turning your fitness routine into a fulfilling journey of self-improvement.

Building confidence with small victories.

Building confidence with small victories is about recognizing and celebrating the progress you make, no matter how small it may seem. For seniors, who may face physical limitations or initial challenges when starting a fitness program, these victories are crucial for cultivating a positive mindset and sustained motivation. The concept of small victories is grounded in the idea that each step forward, no matter how minor, contributes to your overall success. It's about breaking down larger goals into manageable parts and achieving them one by one. For instance, if your goal is to improve balance, a small victory might be successfully standing on one leg for a few seconds without support. This small achievement, while seemingly simple, represents a tangible step toward your larger goal and boosts your confidence.

Each small victory is an opportunity to acknowledge and reward yourself. It's about recognizing that these accomplishments are hard-earned and meaningful. They serve as reminders that you are capable of progress and that you can overcome obstacles. By celebrating these wins, you build a sense of accomplishment that is essential for long-term motivation. It's easy to overlook small successes in favor of a singular focus on the end goal, but acknowledging them is an important part of the journey. Whether it's mastering a new exercise technique, noticing improved flexibility, or simply feeling more comfortable with physical activity, each victory contributes to a more confident and empowered you.

These small victories also provide momentum for tackling bigger challenges. They create a positive feedback loop where each success fuels the desire for more. When you build confidence through small wins, you develop a can-do attitude that makes it easier to face and overcome larger fitness goals. It becomes less about proving something to yourself and more about enjoying the process of improvement. Over time, as you accumulate these victories, they become stepping stones to even greater achievements. The confidence you gain from each small win can be transformative, helping you approach each workout with a positive mindset and the belief that you can achieve more. Building confidence through small victories is not just about the physical gains; it's also about cultivating a resilient, determined spirit that empowers you to live life fully and embrace new challenges with enthusiasm.

Equipment Basics

When it comes to strength training, choosing the right equipment is crucial to ensure both safety and effectiveness. There's a wide range of options available, from resistance bands and dumbbells to household items that can be adapted for strength training. The key is to find what works best for you and aligns with your fitness goals. Resistance bands are a popular choice because they are versatile, lightweight, and easy to use. They provide resistance throughout the range of motion, which can help build muscle strength and improve flexibility. When selecting resistance bands, consider the level of resistance that matches your current strength level. If you're just starting, choose lighter bands to minimize strain and allow for proper form. As you gain strength, you can progress to bands with more resistance to continue challenging your muscles.

Choosing the right equipment: bands, dumbbells, and more.

When it comes to strength training, selecting the right equipment can make a significant difference in your overall experience and effectiveness. The equipment you choose should align with your fitness goals, strength level, and physical condition. Resistance bands are an excellent starting point for many seniors because they are versatile and adaptable. They come in various resistance levels, allowing you to choose one that matches your strength and gradually increase the intensity as you get stronger. Bands are also portable and easy to store, making them ideal for home use or traveling. When choosing resistance bands, look for a set that includes different resistance levels or a pack that allows you to mix and match depending on the exercise. Start with lighter bands if you're a beginner or have limited strength, as they provide a lower level of resistance, which can help prevent injury and allow you to maintain proper form. As you progress, you can move to bands with more resistance to continue challenging your muscles and making gains.

Dumbbells offer a more direct form of resistance and are great for targeting specific muscle groups. They come in various weights, typically ranging from 1 to 50 pounds or more, allowing you to select the appropriate weight based on your strength level. When choosing dumbbells, consider your current fitness level and any pre-existing joint or muscle conditions. A good starting point is a set of adjustable dumbbells that can be easily modified as your strength increases. Adjustable dumbbells allow you to change the weight by adding or removing plates, which can be particularly useful if you're unsure of your exact strength level or want to progress gradually. It's essential to maintain proper posture and ergonomics while using dumbbells to prevent strain or injury. Ensure that your wrists, elbows, and shoulders are in alignment and that you're using a weight that allows you to perform the exercises with good form. If you're not confident in your form, consider consulting a fitness professional who can guide you through proper techniques.

In addition to resistance bands and dumbbells, there are other pieces of equipment that can enhance your strength training routine. Kettlebells, stability balls, medicine balls, and ankle weights are also great options, each offering unique benefits. Kettlebells, for instance, are excellent for functional training and engaging multiple muscle groups simultaneously. Stability balls can improve balance, coordination, and core strength, making them a great addition to your routine as you age. Medicine balls provide an additional challenge for muscle endurance and coordination. Ankle weights can be used for lower body exercises like leg raises or walking to add resistance and strengthen muscles in the legs and hips. The key to choosing the right equipment is to consider what best suits your individual needs, preferences, and goals. The most important thing is to find tools that support proper form, ensure safety, and provide effective resistance as you progress in your fitness journey.

Ensuring proper posture and ergonomics.

Ensuring proper posture and ergonomics is crucial for safe and effective strength training, especially for seniors who may be more susceptible to injury or discomfort. Good posture not only helps prevent strain and overexertion but also maximizes the benefits of your exercises. When performing any exercise, whether it's using resistance bands, dumbbells, or bodyweight movements, it's important to maintain a neutral spine and keep your body in alignment. This means keeping your shoulders relaxed, avoiding rounding your back, and aligning your joints—especially the wrists, elbows, and shoulders—to prevent undue stress on them. Poor posture can lead to discomfort and decrease the effectiveness of your workouts, so it's essential to pay attention to your form during every movement.

Ergonomics also play a significant role in protecting your body from injury.

Ergonomic principles involve designing equipment, workspaces, and routines that fit your body's natural mechanics and support a healthy posture. When using equipment like dumbbells, resistance bands, or household items, make sure they are positioned at a comfortable height and distance from your body. For example, when lifting dumbbells, hold them close to your body to minimize strain on your back and shoulders. Avoid any movements that require you to bend excessively or reach out too far. This helps reduce the risk of injury and allows you to maintain control over the weight or resistance.

Additionally, paying attention to how you transition between exercises is important. Moving smoothly from one exercise to the next without jerky or abrupt movements ensures that you maintain control and alignment throughout the routine. It's also a good idea to take short breaks between sets to reset your posture, especially if you're using heavier weights or more intense resistance. Adjust your grip, stance, or seating position as needed to ensure that your body remains in a stable, comfortable position. The goal is to minimize the risk of injury and maximize the effectiveness of each exercise. By focusing on proper posture and ergonomics, you can train more efficiently and with greater safety, making strength training a sustainable part of your fitness routine as you age.

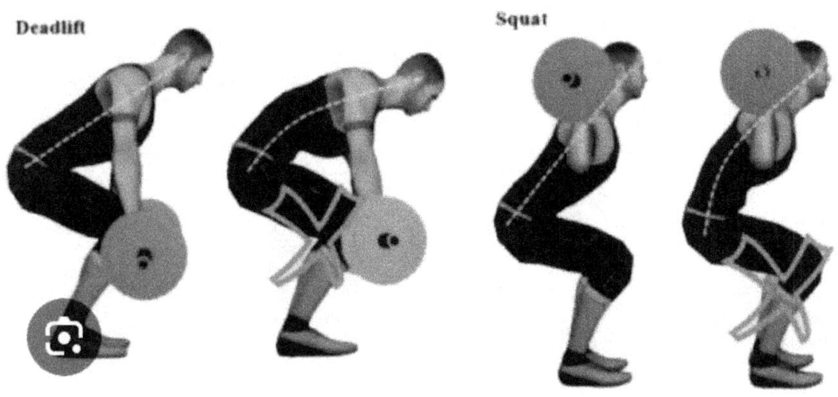

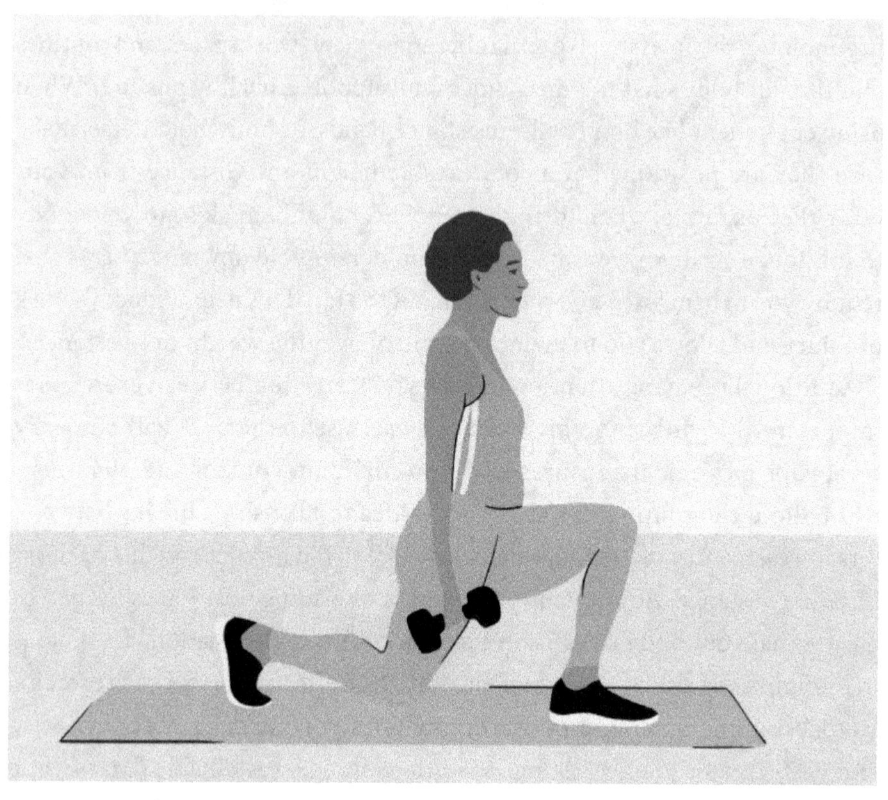

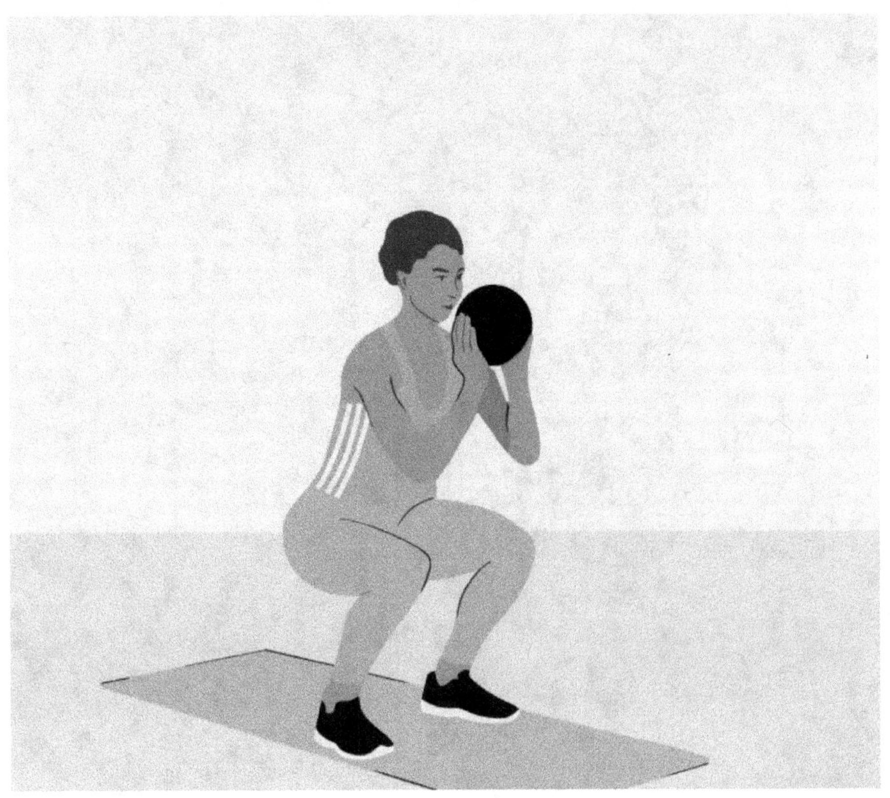

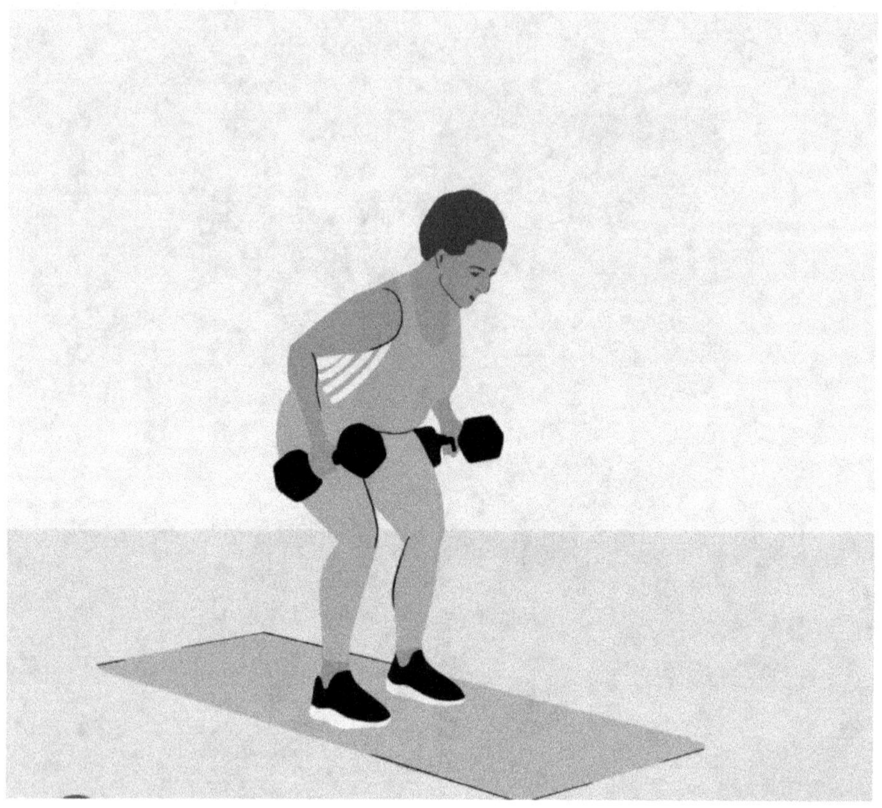

Adapting household items for strength training.

Adapting household items for strength training is a practical and cost-effective way to get started with exercises that improve muscle strength and endurance. The beauty of using everyday items is that they can easily be incorporated into your fitness routine without requiring a significant financial investment in specialized equipment. Water bottles, cans of food, bags of rice, or even books and newspapers can serve as makeshift weights for resistance exercises. This not only makes strength training accessible but also allows you to perform a wide range of exercises that target different muscle groups effectively. The key is to choose items that provide some resistance and are safe to handle without straining your muscles or joints.

When selecting household items for strength training, consider their weight, stability, and safety. For instance, a full water bottle or a can of beans can be used for exercises like bicep curls, shoulder presses, or chest presses. These items offer a similar level of resistance as dumbbells but at a lower cost. It's important to ensure that whatever you use can be comfortably lifted without compromising your form or risking injury. Start with lighter weights to allow your body to adapt, and gradually increase the load as your strength improves. If an item feels too heavy or unwieldy, look for alternatives or adjust the amount of weight in a safe and controlled manner.

In addition to weight, consider the ergonomics of your makeshift equipment. Ensure that they have a secure grip and are free from sharp edges or unstable bases that could pose a safety risk. Items like a sturdy chair or a step can also be used as platforms for exercises like tricep dips or step-ups, providing resistance and supporting balance. Adapting household items for strength training allows you to make use of what you already have, minimizing the need for a dedicated gym or extensive purchases. It's about getting creative with what's available and turning ordinary objects into tools for building strength and enhancing your fitness. This approach not only saves money but also makes strength training convenient and adaptable to any space—whether at home, in a park, or during travel.

4

Chapter 3: Core Principles of Strength Training for Seniors

Frequency and Duration

When it comes to strength training for seniors, determining the right frequency and duration of exercise is crucial for achieving optimal results. The goal is to find a balance between consistent activity and adequate rest to allow your body to recover and adapt. For most older adults, a good starting point is two to three sessions per week, each lasting around 30 to 45 minutes. This allows you to focus on different muscle groups in each session and provides enough time for your body to recover in between workouts. The key is to gradually increase the intensity and duration of your workouts as your strength and endurance improve. Starting slowly and progressing gradually is essential to avoid overtraining and reduce the risk of injury.

How often to exercise for optimal results.

When it comes to determining how often to exercise for optimal results, there's no one-size-fits-all answer, as it largely depends on your individual fitness level, goals, and health status. For seniors aiming to improve muscle strength, maintain mobility, and boost overall health, a moderate approach works best. Generally, aiming for two to three strength training sessions per week is a solid starting point. Each session should focus on different muscle groups to allow each set of muscles enough time to recover before being worked again. This frequency helps to maintain muscle mass, increase endurance, and enhance overall functional fitness.

Strength training at this frequency also allows you to incorporate variation in your routine. This means you can target different muscle groups on different days—like focusing on your upper body one day, your lower body the next, and a full-body workout on another. By alternating the muscle groups you train, you prevent overuse injuries and ensure that all muscles have adequate time to rebuild and strengthen between sessions. This approach also helps to keep the workouts engaging, as you're not constantly working the same muscles, which can lead to boredom or burnout.

If you're just starting out or have been inactive for a while, it's wise to begin with less frequent sessions—perhaps two times a week—to allow your body to adapt. As you build strength and endurance, you can gradually increase the frequency. Some seniors may benefit from additional workouts if they are specifically working towards improving athletic performance or have specific health goals, but it's important to do so gradually and not at the expense of proper recovery. Listen to your body and adjust your routine based on how you feel. If you're overly fatigued, have soreness that doesn't improve with rest, or notice any discomfort, it might be an indication that your body needs more time to recover. The goal is to find a balance that supports consistent progress while keeping injury risks low.

Balancing rest and activity for recovery.

Balancing rest and activity is crucial for recovery and overall well-being, especially in strength training for seniors. Recovery is not just about taking breaks between exercises; it's a holistic process that involves rest days, sleep, nutrition, and light physical activity. When you engage in strength training, you place stress on your muscles, which causes microscopic tears and leads to muscle growth and strength improvement over time. However, these muscles need time to repair and rebuild. This is where rest comes into play.

Adequate rest days—typically at least 48 hours between workouts targeting the same muscle group—are essential to allow your body to recover fully. During rest, your body releases growth hormone, which is crucial for repairing and rebuilding muscle tissue. It's also when inflammation and muscle soreness are minimized, making way for increased strength and endurance. Without sufficient rest, you risk overtraining, which can lead to fatigue, decreased performance, and an increased likelihood of injury.

In addition to scheduled rest days, incorporating light physical activity can aid recovery. Activities such as walking, swimming, or gentle stretching can help improve circulation, which facilitates nutrient delivery to muscles and helps flush out metabolic byproducts like lactic acid that build up during exercise. These low-intensity activities are a great way to keep active without adding stress to already taxed muscles. They also serve to maintain mobility and keep the joints lubricated, reducing stiffness and promoting overall flexibility.

Nutrition plays a vital role in recovery as well. Consuming a balanced diet with adequate protein is important for muscle repair. Protein provides the amino acids necessary for muscle repair and growth, so including lean meats, fish, eggs, dairy, legumes, and plant-based protein sources in your diet can support recovery. Carbohydrates are equally important as they replenish glycogen stores in muscles and provide the energy needed for effective workouts. Healthy fats contribute to overall cellular health and hormone production, which also support muscle growth and recovery.

Monitoring your body's signals is key to balancing rest and activity. If you feel overly fatigued, sore, or notice a decline in performance, it's a sign that your body needs more time to rest. On the other hand, if you're feeling energetic and your muscles are feeling strong, a light activity session could be beneficial to maintain circulation and keep your body moving. The goal is to find a balance that supports steady progress and prevents setbacks due to overexertion.

Structuring a weekly fitness plan.

Structuring a weekly fitness plan is about creating a balanced routine that supports your fitness goals and ensures you're working all major muscle groups without overtraining. A well-structured plan takes into account frequency, duration, intensity, and variety. For seniors, this plan should be adaptable and cater to individual capabilities and progress over time. The aim is to create a schedule that's both sustainable and enjoyable, making fitness a regular part of your week that's not only beneficial but also manageable.

Start by deciding how many days per week you want to dedicate to strength training. Two to three days is typically a good range for seniors starting out, but this can be adjusted based on your fitness level and recovery needs. Once you've established the frequency, you can divide your workouts across the week. For instance, if you decide on three days of strength training, you might split it into two upper body days and one lower body day, or have a full-body workout on each session. This distribution helps target different muscle groups on different days, allowing each set of muscles sufficient recovery time between sessions.

In addition to strength training, your weekly plan should also include flexibility exercises, balance training, and cardiovascular activity. Flexibility exercises, such as yoga or gentle stretching, can help maintain joint health and prevent stiffness. Balance exercises are important for improving stability and reducing the risk of falls—a critical consideration as you age. Cardiovascular activities like walking, swimming, or cycling should complement your strength workouts to improve heart health, endurance, and overall energy levels. These activities also help burn calories, manage weight, and keep you active outside of dedicated strength training sessions.

Setting specific, achievable goals for each session can make the plan more effective. For instance, you might aim to increase the number of repetitions, the weight lifted, or the number of sets completed over time. This progression ensures you're consistently challenging your muscles and making steady progress without overexertion. Your weekly plan should also include adequate rest days—typically one to two days per week—where you focus on recovery through light activity or complete rest. These rest days are crucial for muscle repair and injury prevention.

Lastly, monitor your progress by tracking workouts and adjusting the plan as needed. This could mean modifying exercises, changing the order of workouts, or altering the intensity to match your current fitness level. Pay attention to how your body feels and be open to adjusting the plan to meet your needs. A flexible approach allows you to fine-tune the routine over time, ensuring that it remains effective and sustainable as you progress in your strength training journey. The key to structuring a weekly fitness plan is to make it realistic, enjoyable, and aligned with your long-term goals, so you can maintain consistency and enjoy the benefits of a strong, active lifestyle.

Intensity and Progression

When it comes to intensity and progression in strength training, especially for seniors, it's important to start slowly and gradually build up. Begin with low-intensity workouts that focus on basic movements and light weights. This helps to familiarize your body with the exercises and reduces the risk of injury. It's not about going hard from the start; it's about creating a foundation that will support long-term gains in strength and endurance. Starting slowly also allows you to pay attention to proper form and posture, which are crucial for avoiding strain and overexertion.

Starting with low-intensity workouts.

Starting with low-intensity workouts is a fundamental approach, especially for seniors, as it sets the stage for a safe and effective strength training routine. The objective here is to introduce exercise in a way that is gentle on the body, minimizes injury risks, and allows you to build up gradually. Low-intensity workouts are essentially the basics—simple movements with light weights, bodyweight exercises, or resistance bands that don't put excessive strain on your muscles or joints. This introductory phase is all about learning proper form and technique, ensuring you understand the mechanics of each exercise before progressing to more challenging levels.

Low-intensity workouts are ideal for seniors because they help you build a foundational strength without overloading your system. They can include exercises like seated leg lifts, gentle squats, arm curls with light dumbbells, or even simple yoga poses. These movements allow you to engage muscles and improve flexibility without placing undue stress on your body. By starting low and slow, you also give your body the chance to adapt to the physical demands of exercise. This adaptability is particularly important as aging bodies may have reduced tolerance for vigorous activity.

The beauty of low-intensity workouts is that they lay the groundwork for further progression. As you grow more comfortable with the basic exercises and notice improvements in strength and endurance, you can gradually begin to add more intensity. This could mean increasing the weight, adding more repetitions, or exploring more challenging exercises that target different muscle groups. The key is to maintain a steady pace, allowing your body to strengthen and recover properly between sessions. It's about building a safe and sustainable fitness routine that respects your limits while still encouraging growth. Starting low-intensity workouts also provides an opportunity to monitor your body's responses to exercise, making it easier to identify any discomfort or signs that you may be overexerting yourself. This approach helps ensure that you are progressing at a healthy rate, preventing injuries and promoting long-term fitness success.

Gradually increasing resistance and repetitions.

Gradually increasing resistance and repetitions is a key strategy in strength training that allows you to safely challenge your muscles without risking injury. This method is all about progression—slowly and consistently building up the difficulty of your workouts as your body adapts and gets stronger. By doing so, you stimulate muscle growth and endurance, which is essential for maintaining strength as you age. The process involves increasing the amount of weight, the number of sets, or the number of repetitions you perform over time. This gradual approach ensures that your body can keep up with the increased demand without becoming overly fatigued or strained.

Start by selecting weights or resistance levels that are light enough to allow you to complete the exercises with good form. This ensures that you're engaging the right muscles and reduces the risk of injury. Once you feel comfortable with the exercise and can perform a set with good technique, you can begin to increase the resistance. This could mean adding more weight to your dumbbells, moving up a resistance band level, or adjusting the incline or speed on a piece of exercise equipment. The goal is to make your muscles work harder, which encourages growth and strength improvements.

As you increase resistance, you also need to adjust the number of repetitions and sets accordingly. Initially, aim for a moderate number of repetitions (typically 8-12) and sets (2-3) that allow you to maintain proper form throughout. Once these repetitions become easier, you can start to gradually increase the number. This might mean adding a few more repetitions to each set, increasing the number of sets, or both. The idea is to continue challenging your muscles, pushing them beyond their comfort zone. Over time, this will help improve muscle endurance and strength, which are critical for maintaining physical function and reducing the risk of injury as you age.

Recognizing the signs that indicate you're ready to increase resistance or repetitions is important. These signs include feeling like the exercise is getting too easy, completing sets without feeling fatigued, or being able to perform movements with perfect form and minimal effort. When you notice these indicators, it's time to push yourself a bit harder by adding more resistance or increasing the number of repetitions. However, the increase should be gradual and aligned with your body's capacity to adapt. Sudden jumps in intensity can lead to muscle strain, fatigue, or setbacks. It's all about finding the right balance that allows for continuous progress without compromising your safety and well-being.

Recognizing when to adjust your routine.

Recognizing when to adjust your routine is a critical aspect of strength training that ensures you're continually progressing in a safe and effective manner. This involves listening to your body's signals and making informed changes based on how you're feeling physically and mentally. It's about understanding when to dial back the intensity, modify exercises, or take a break altogether. Adjusting your routine is not about giving up; it's a smart way to optimize your training and prevent overtraining, injuries, or plateaus. The goal is to maintain a balance that challenges your muscles without pushing them beyond their limits.

There are several indicators that suggest it might be time to tweak your routine. These can include persistent fatigue, joint pain, discomfort, or a lack of improvement despite consistent effort. If you find that certain exercises cause pain or exacerbate existing injuries, it's a sign that those movements need to be altered or replaced with alternatives that are safer for your body. Similarly, if you're not seeing the progress you expect—such as a plateau in muscle strength or endurance—it might be an indication that you need to change things up. This could involve adjusting the weight, changing the number of repetitions, altering the frequency of workouts, or incorporating new exercises to stimulate muscle growth in different ways.

Another important factor to consider is the recovery phase. If you're not giving your muscles adequate time to heal and repair, they won't grow stronger. This is particularly true as we age, when recovery takes longer. If you're feeling unusually sore or fatigued, it's a sign that you might need more rest days between sessions or lighter workouts. Adjusting your routine based on recovery needs helps prevent burnout and keeps your motivation levels high. You might also need to reconsider the overall structure of your workouts—switching from a high-intensity plan to a more moderate one if your body isn't coping well. This flexibility is key to long-term success, allowing you to adapt your fitness goals to fit your current physical state.

Lastly, setting realistic and achievable benchmarks is crucial. As you progress, the goals you initially set might become less relevant or achievable if your body changes or if you experience new health challenges. This might mean scaling back expectations or redefining your targets to better align with your current capabilities and objectives. Recognizing when to adjust your routine is about being proactive and responsive to your body's needs. It's a continuous process of assessment, reflection, and adjustment that ensures your strength training is sustainable and effective over the long term.

Key Focus Areas

When it comes to strength training for seniors, the focus should be on more than just building muscle. It's about enhancing overall physical function and quality of life. Strengthening major muscle groups is crucial because it supports basic movements like walking, climbing stairs, and getting in and out of chairs. These are the functional movements that matter most for daily living. By targeting the muscles in your legs, arms, back, and core, you not only improve strength but also help prevent falls and injuries. A strong foundation reduces the risk of common age-related issues like osteoporosis and arthritis.

Strengthening major muscle groups.

Strengthening major muscle groups is a foundational aspect of any effective strength training program, particularly for seniors over 60. This focus is about ensuring that the body's primary muscles—those that support movement, balance, and overall physical function—are robust enough to handle daily activities and unexpected physical challenges. Major muscle groups include the quadriceps, hamstrings, calves, chest, back, shoulders, and arms. By targeting these areas, you improve overall body strength, which is crucial for maintaining mobility, preventing falls, and reducing the risk of injury. A well-rounded approach ensures that no muscle group is left behind, which helps maintain harmony in physical movements and contributes to a balanced and efficient body.

Strengthening these muscle groups goes beyond aesthetics; it's about functionality and health. For instance, strong leg muscles are essential for walking, climbing stairs, and maintaining balance. They help propel you forward and provide stability when navigating uneven surfaces. The core muscles—comprising the abdominals, lower back, and obliques—are crucial for maintaining good posture and transferring power from the upper body to the lower body, as well as for protecting the spine during daily activities. Similarly, strengthening the chest, back, and shoulder muscles supports activities like lifting, pushing, and pulling—whether it's loading groceries into the car or carrying laundry up the stairs.

Including exercises that target these muscle groups can be done using weights, resistance bands, or bodyweight exercises. For example, squats and lunges are excellent for strengthening the legs, while push-ups and shoulder presses help build upper body strength. Deadlifts and bent-over rows are great for targeting the back and core, promoting good posture and spine health. By incorporating a variety of exercises, you ensure that all major muscle groups are adequately challenged and strengthened. This balanced approach not only enhances your physical capacity but also reduces the risk of muscle imbalances, which can lead to injury and limit functional movement. A strong body is better equipped to withstand the demands of daily life and supports overall well-being as you age.

Emphasizing balance, stability, and coordination.

Emphasizing balance, stability, and coordination in a strength training program is particularly important for seniors over 60 because these elements are directly linked to fall prevention and overall functional independence. Balance refers to the ability to maintain your center of gravity over your base of support, whether you're standing still or moving. Stability involves the body's ability to maintain equilibrium and posture under various conditions, such as shifting weight from one leg to another. Coordination is the smooth integration of various muscle groups to perform complex movements without stumbling or awkwardness. Strength training exercises that target these areas can help seniors move more freely, confidently, and safely, reducing the risk of falls and injuries.

Balance exercises are designed to challenge your body's proprioceptive system—your sense of where your body is in space. Activities like standing on one leg, using a balance board, or walking in a figure-eight pattern improve proprioception and teach your muscles how to respond to changes in movement or posture. These exercises can be performed with minimal equipment and at home, making them accessible even for those with limited mobility. As your balance improves, so does your ability to react quickly and maintain control during everyday activities like bending down, reaching for items, or simply standing up from a chair.

Stability exercises strengthen the core and the muscles around the joints, particularly the ankles, knees, and hips, which are key areas for maintaining balance and reducing injury risk. Exercises like seated leg lifts, heel-to-toe walks, and wall push-ups help in building a stable base, which is critical for safe movement and functional independence. These exercises can also be adapted to accommodate different levels of fitness and physical limitations, ensuring they are appropriate for all seniors, regardless of their starting point.

Coordination exercises, on the other hand, enhance the ability of your brain and body to work together. Activities that require you to move different parts of your body simultaneously—such as walking while carrying weights, following a set of simple dance steps, or doing arm circles while balancing on one foot—help train the brain to integrate movement patterns effectively. Improved coordination can make daily tasks easier and reduce the risk of tripping or losing balance. By integrating these exercises into your routine, you're not just building muscle strength but also fostering an agile and responsive body that can handle the challenges of aging.

Prioritizing functional movements for daily tasks.

Prioritizing functional movements for daily tasks is about tailoring strength training exercises to replicate real-life activities that seniors perform regularly. Functional movements are the types of actions that allow you to live independently and safely, such as getting in and out of a chair, bending over to tie your shoes, lifting a grocery bag, or reaching up to a high shelf. These exercises aim to maintain, enhance, and restore the physical skills needed to manage daily life without requiring assistance. By prioritizing these functional movements in your strength training routine, you can ensure that you are building strength and endurance in a way that directly translates to better quality of life.

Functional exercises challenge your body to work as an integrated unit. For instance, squats mimic sitting down and standing up from a chair, which are actions that you perform many times a day. Similarly, exercises like lunges simulate stepping over an obstacle or getting up off the floor after a fall. By practicing these movements with proper form and resistance, you strengthen the muscles that support them, thereby reducing the risk of injury and making these tasks easier to perform. The goal is to make everyday activities as effortless and safe as possible, which helps maintain independence and reduces the fear of falling or losing mobility as you age.

Additionally, prioritizing functional movements can improve overall body mechanics and movement efficiency. These exercises not only build strength but also promote better posture and alignment, which can alleviate aches and pains often associated with aging. For instance, lifting weights overhead in a controlled manner can strengthen the shoulder and upper back muscles, which are essential for reaching high shelves and hanging curtains. Similarly, exercises like carrying weights while walking help simulate carrying groceries, which strengthens the grip and shoulder muscles while also improving cardiovascular fitness. By integrating these exercises into your routine, you create a well-rounded training program that supports both the specific physical demands of daily life and long-term health.

5

Chapter 4: Building Strength Safely with Bodyweight Exercises

Upper Body Strength

When it comes to maintaining upper body strength, it's important to focus on exercises that target the arms, shoulders, and chest muscles. Wall push-ups are an excellent way to strengthen the arm and chest muscles without requiring you to lift your full body weight. By placing your hands against a sturdy wall at shoulder height, you can perform a push-up motion, which engages the pectoral muscles and the front deltoids. This exercise is particularly beneficial because it can be easily modified for different levels of strength—whether you need to start with a more inclined position or gradually progress to a full push-up.

Wall push-ups for arm and chest muscles.

Wall push-ups are a simplified variation of the traditional push-up that make it easier to strengthen the arm and chest muscles without putting too much strain on the body, making them ideal for seniors over 60 with limited endurance or who are just starting out with strength training. To perform a wall push-up, you stand facing a sturdy wall with your hands placed flat against it at shoulder height. Your feet should be a comfortable distance away from the wall, providing a stable base. From this position, you bend your elbows and slowly lower your body towards the wall, keeping your body in a straight line from head to heels.

This exercise effectively targets the pectoral muscles (chest), the anterior deltoids (front shoulders), and the triceps (back of the arms). By leaning into the wall and pushing away, you work against gravity, which strengthens these key muscle groups. Wall push-ups can be modified to suit your fitness level— if needed, you can start with a more inclined position where your hands are higher than shoulder height, which reduces the amount of body weight you have to lift. As you progress, you can lower your hands gradually, until you're able to perform a full push-up against the wall, and eventually transition to standard push-ups on the floor as your strength improves.

Wall push-ups are particularly beneficial for seniors because they help build muscle strength in the upper body, which is crucial for maintaining good posture, supporting arm movements, and preventing injuries. They also improve upper body endurance, making it easier to perform everyday activities like reaching for objects on high shelves or pushing yourself up from a seated position. By incorporating wall push-ups into your routine, you can strengthen the muscles involved in these actions, which in turn enhances your overall functional fitness and boosts your confidence in performing daily tasks.

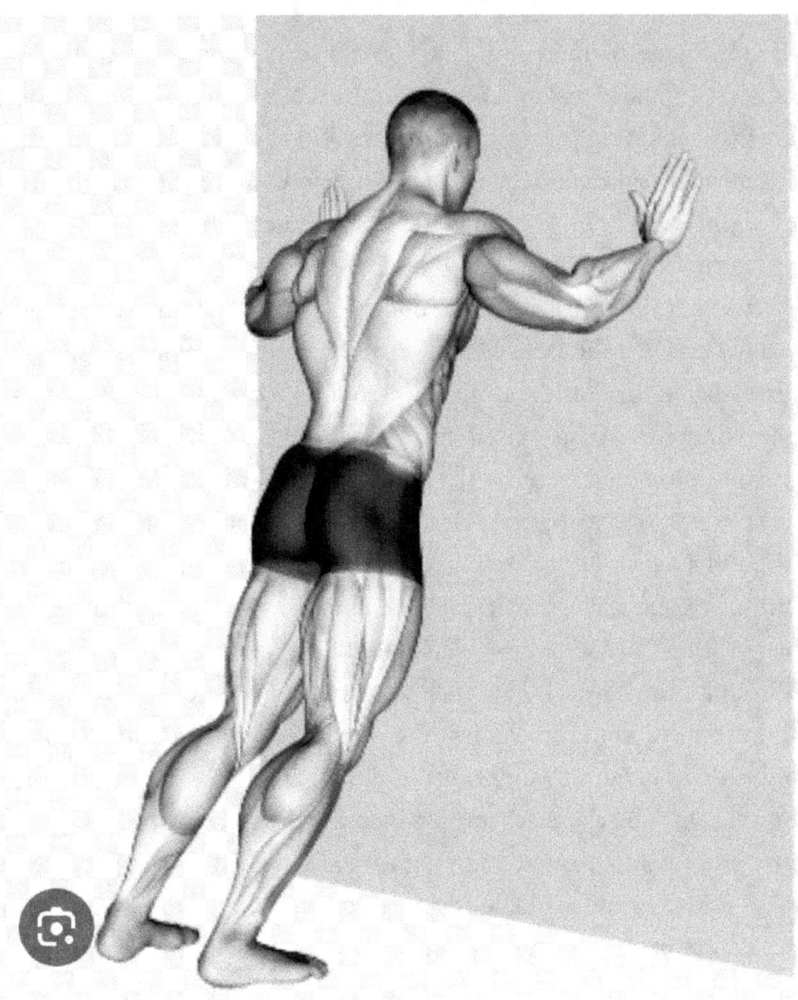

Seated arm raises for shoulders.

Seated arm raises are a straightforward yet effective exercise designed to target the shoulder muscles, making them an excellent choice for seniors over 60 who want to improve their shoulder strength and mobility. This exercise can be performed while sitting in a sturdy chair, which not only ensures safety but also makes it accessible for those with limited mobility or who are just beginning their fitness journey. To perform seated arm raises, sit upright with your feet flat on the ground and your back straight. Hold a pair of light dumbbells or even water bottles in each hand, depending on your strength level.

To start, extend your arms straight out to the sides at shoulder height. Lift your arms slowly to shoulder height, keeping your movements controlled and steady. Hold for a brief moment at the top before lowering them back down to your sides. This simple movement engages the deltoid muscles, which are located on the top of the shoulders, and works them through a full range of motion. Seated arm raises are not just about building strength; they also enhance shoulder stability, improve posture, and increase range of motion, which can be particularly beneficial as we age and the risk of shoulder stiffness and weakness increases.

This exercise can be easily modified to match your current fitness level. If you find the movement too challenging, you can start with a smaller range of motion or reduce the weight of the dumbbells. As you become more comfortable with the exercise, you can increase the weight or repetitions to continue progressing. Seated arm raises are also a great way to prepare the shoulders for other more challenging exercises, as they help warm up the muscles and improve blood flow, reducing the risk of injury during other strength training activities. By incorporating seated arm raises into your fitness routine, you're not only working towards stronger shoulders but also fostering better overall shoulder health, which is essential for maintaining functional independence and performing daily tasks with ease.

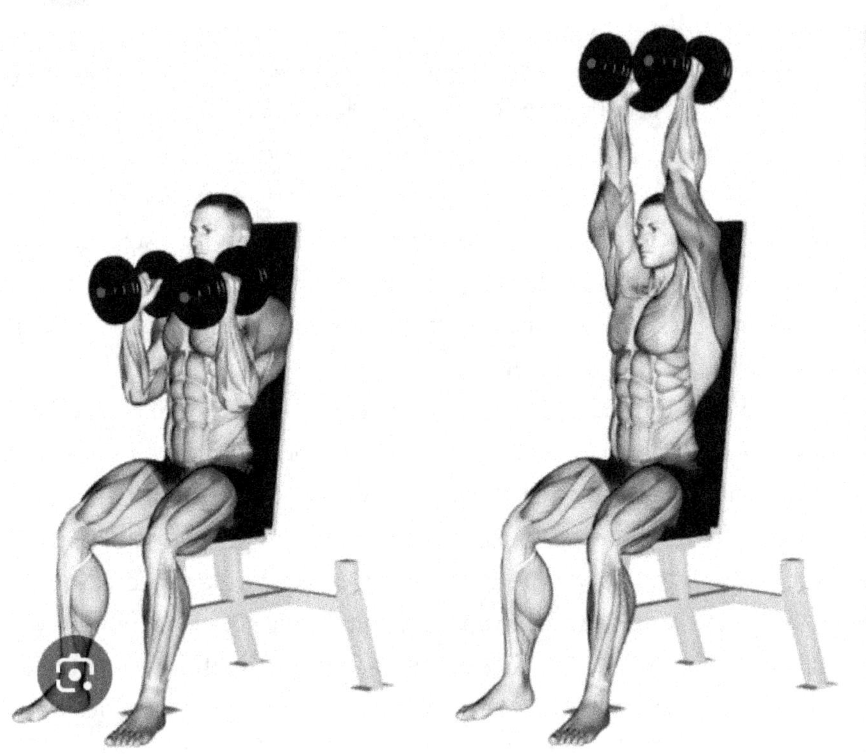

Chair dips for triceps.

Chair dips are an effective exercise for targeting the triceps—the muscles located at the back of the upper arm. This exercise can be performed using a sturdy chair, making it a convenient option for seniors over 60 who want to improve arm strength and tone. To perform chair dips, start by sitting on the edge of a stable chair with your hands placed on the seat just beside your hips. Your fingers should be pointing forward, and your feet should be flat on the floor, with knees bent at a comfortable angle. From this position, gently lift your body off the chair and move your buttocks forward, balancing on your palms.

To begin the exercise, slowly bend your elbows and lower your body towards the floor, keeping your upper arms close to your body. Lower until your elbows are at a 90-degree angle, then press through your palms to push yourself back up to the starting position. This controlled movement strengthens the triceps muscles, which are crucial for arm strength and stability. Chair dips are particularly beneficial for improving arm tone and definition, making them an excellent choice for seniors who want to enhance their appearance and functionality.

For those with limited endurance or strength, chair dips can be modified to make them more accessible. You can adjust the difficulty by extending your legs out in front of you or placing your feet on the floor with knees bent. You can also start with fewer repetitions and gradually increase as you build strength. As you perform this exercise regularly, you'll notice improvements not only in tricep strength but also in shoulder stability and overall arm endurance. Chair dips can be incorporated into a well-rounded upper body workout routine, helping seniors maintain strength and flexibility in their arms, which is essential for daily activities such as carrying groceries, reaching, and pushing.

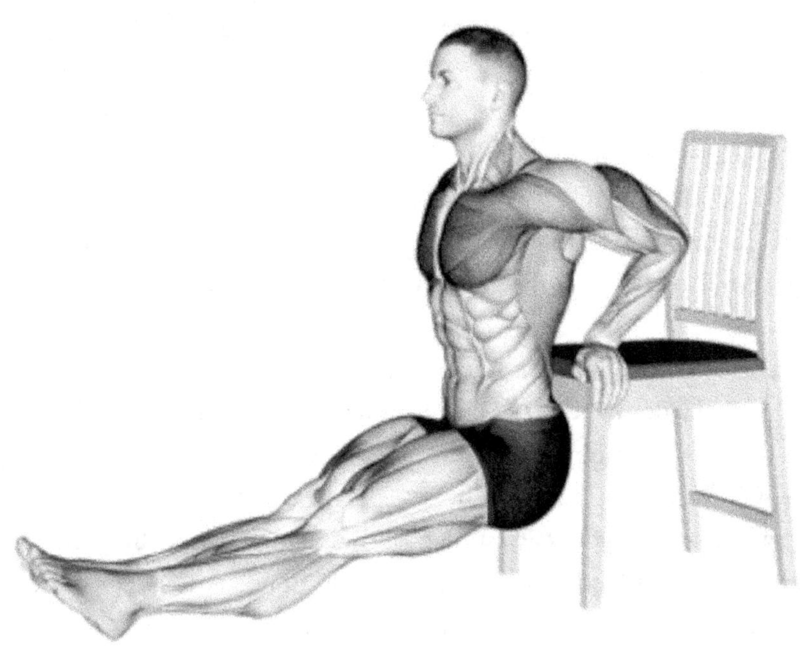

Core and Back Strength

Building strength in the core and back is essential for maintaining stability, balance, and posture, especially as we age. The core serves as the foundation for nearly every movement we perform, and a strong back supports the spine, reducing the risk of injury and improving overall mobility. By focusing on exercises that target these areas, seniors over 60 can enhance their functional fitness and enjoy greater independence in their daily lives.

Seated knee lifts for abdominal engagement.

Seated knee lifts are a simple yet highly effective exercise for engaging the abdominal muscles, making them an excellent choice for seniors seeking to strengthen their core in a safe and controlled manner. This exercise can be performed while seated in a sturdy chair, ensuring stability and minimizing the risk of strain or injury. It is particularly beneficial for individuals with limited endurance or mobility, as it provides a low-impact way to target the core muscles, which play a vital role in balance, posture, and functional movement.

To perform seated knee lifts, sit upright on the edge of a chair with your feet flat on the floor and your hands gripping the sides of the seat for support. Engage your abdominal muscles by drawing your belly button toward your spine, which helps protect the lower back. Slowly lift one knee toward your chest while keeping your back straight and avoiding any slouching. Lower the leg back down with control and repeat on the opposite side. For those with more strength and stability, lifting both knees simultaneously can increase the intensity of the exercise and further challenge the core.

This movement specifically activates the lower abdominal muscles, which are often neglected in everyday activities. Strengthening this part of the core improves stability and supports proper posture, reducing the risk of falls and alleviating back discomfort. Additionally, because the exercise requires balance and coordination, it helps train the body for real-life movements, such as getting up from a seated position or stabilizing during unexpected shifts in weight.

Seated knee lifts are versatile and can be adapted to suit different fitness levels. Beginners can start with smaller knee lifts, gradually increasing the range of motion as strength improves. Adding light ankle weights or holding the raised knee in position for a few seconds can also intensify the exercise for those seeking a greater challenge. Regularly incorporating seated knee lifts into a fitness routine can lead to noticeable improvements in abdominal strength, overall core stability, and confidence in performing daily tasks that require balance and coordination.

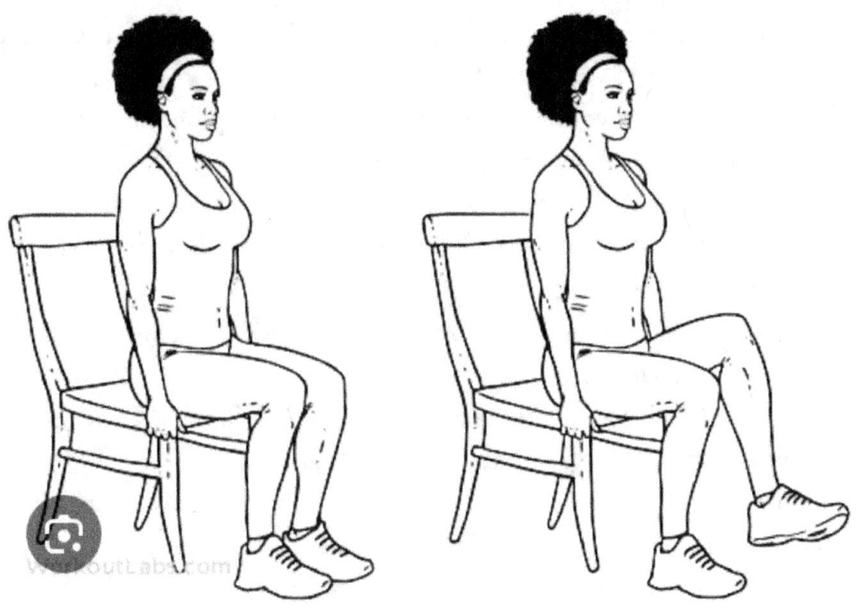

Cat-cow stretches for spinal flexibility.

Cat-cow stretches are a gentle and highly effective exercise for improving spinal flexibility, promoting back health, and reducing stiffness. This dynamic movement, often associated with yoga, alternates between two poses—cat (arching the back upward) and cow (arching the back downward)—to stretch and strengthen the muscles along the spine and surrounding areas. For seniors, particularly those experiencing back tightness or reduced mobility, this exercise can offer a safe and soothing way to maintain spinal health.

To perform cat-cow stretches, you can start either seated on a chair or on your hands and knees on a comfortable surface. For seniors with limited mobility, the seated variation is often more accessible and equally beneficial. In the seated version, sit upright with your feet flat on the floor and hands resting on your knees. Begin by inhaling deeply and arching your back, lifting your chest and tilting your pelvis forward into the cow position. This opens up the spine and engages the lower back muscles. Then, as you exhale, round your back by pulling your belly button inward, tucking your chin toward your chest, and tilting your pelvis backward into the cat position. This gently stretches the muscles along the spine and shoulders.

The movement between these two poses promotes flexibility and mobility in the spine, which is crucial for maintaining a healthy posture and preventing discomfort as we age. Cat-cow stretches also increase blood flow to the spinal discs and muscles, nourishing these critical areas and reducing the risk of stiffness or pain. This exercise can be particularly helpful for seniors dealing with conditions such as arthritis, as it helps loosen tight joints and improve the range of motion without putting undue stress on the body.

In addition to its physical benefits, cat-cow stretches have a calming effect, as the rhythmic breathing and gentle movements can help alleviate stress and tension. Performing this exercise regularly, even for just a few minutes a day, can lead to significant improvements in spinal flexibility, reduced back discomfort, and enhanced overall mobility. For seniors, incorporating cat-cow stretches into their routine is a simple yet powerful way to keep the spine healthy and functional, supporting a more active and comfortable lifestyle.

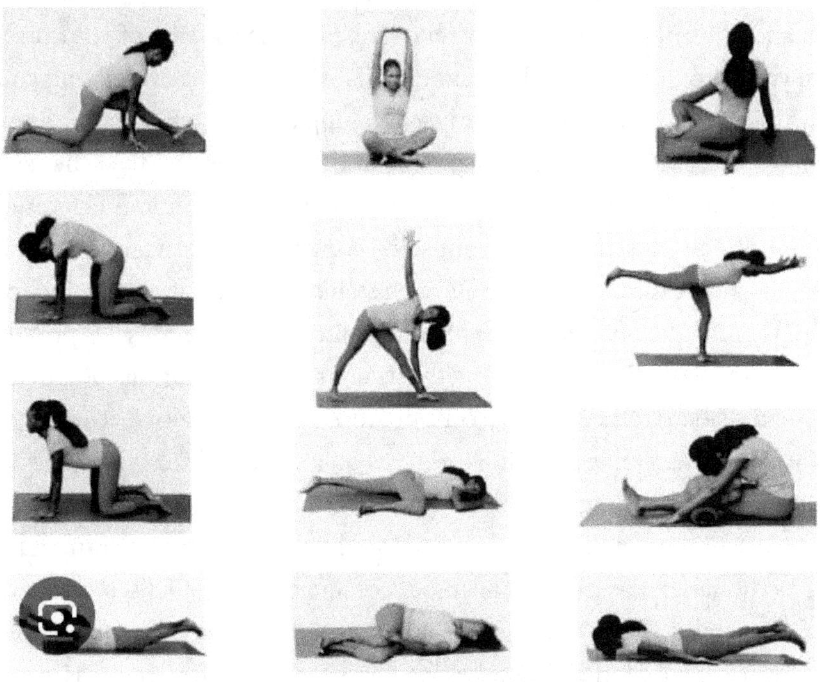

Side stretches for oblique muscles.

Side stretches are an essential exercise for targeting the oblique muscles, which run along the sides of the torso and play a critical role in supporting core strength, balance, and rotational movements. These muscles are often overlooked in traditional fitness routines, but they are vital for everyday activities like reaching, bending, and twisting. For seniors, side stretches offer a gentle and effective way to improve flexibility, reduce stiffness, and maintain functional movement.

To perform a side stretch, sit upright in a sturdy chair or stand with your feet shoulder-width apart for added stability. Start by placing one hand on your hip or holding onto the side of the chair for support. Extend your opposite arm overhead and lean gently to the side, keeping your movements slow and controlled. You should feel a stretch along the side of your torso, from your shoulder to your hip. Avoid collapsing forward or twisting your body; the goal is to lengthen the muscles along the side while maintaining proper posture. Return to the starting position and repeat on the other side.

The primary benefit of side stretches is the elongation and activation of the oblique muscles. These muscles contribute significantly to core strength and are essential for maintaining stability during lateral movements. Strengthening the obliques helps prevent injuries, as these muscles provide critical support to the spine during twisting or bending motions. Regularly practicing side stretches can also improve flexibility, making it easier to perform daily tasks like reaching for items on a shelf or tying your shoes.

Beyond strengthening the obliques, side stretches promote better posture and reduce tension in the shoulders and lower back. As we age, tightness and stiffness in these areas can become more common, leading to discomfort and reduced mobility. Side stretches help counteract these effects by encouraging a greater range of motion and relieving pressure in the affected areas.

For seniors with limited endurance or mobility, side stretches can be easily modified. Performing the movement while seated or reducing the range of motion can still provide significant benefits. Over time, incorporating side stretches into a regular fitness routine can lead to increased flexibility, enhanced core stability, and greater ease in performing everyday movements, contributing to a more active and independent lifestyle.

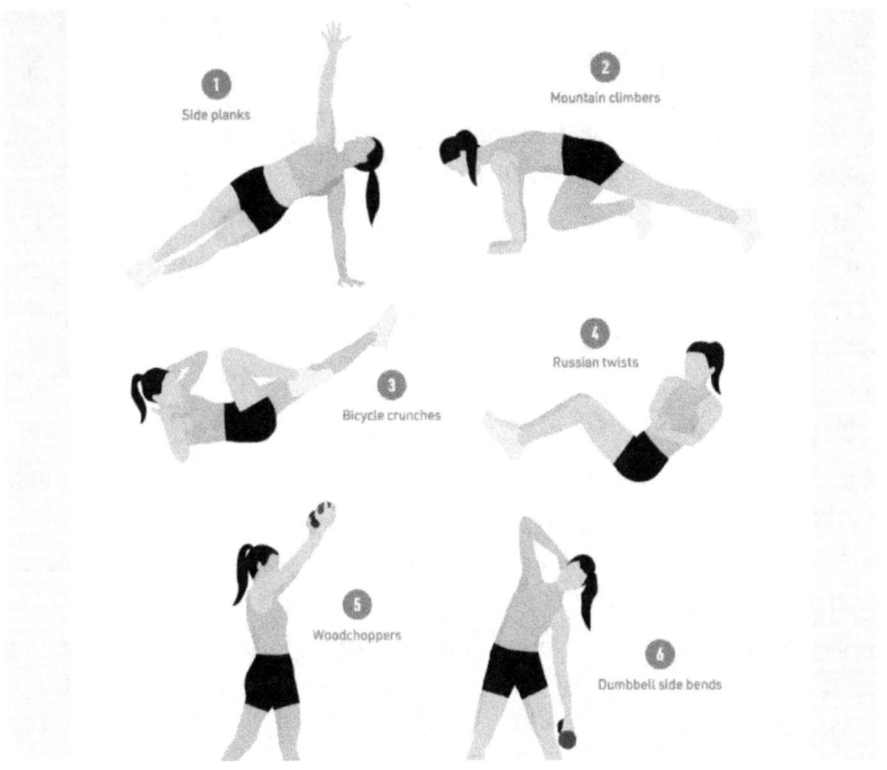

Lower Body Strength

Building lower body strength is essential for maintaining mobility, balance, and independence as we age. The muscles in the legs, hips, and feet are the foundation for many daily activities, from standing up and walking to climbing stairs and navigating uneven terrain. Strengthening these areas not only enhances physical performance but also helps reduce the risk of falls, which are a major concern for older adults. Incorporating specific exercises that target the lower body can lead to significant improvements in overall stability, endurance, and quality of life.

Chair squats for quads and glutes.

Chair squats are a highly effective and practical exercise for strengthening the quadriceps and glutes, two major muscle groups that play a critical role in lower body mobility and stability. For seniors, this movement mimics the functional action of sitting down and standing up, a motion we perform multiple times daily. Incorporating chair squats into a fitness routine can significantly enhance the strength required for these tasks while also improving balance and overall leg endurance.

To perform chair squats, begin by standing in front of a sturdy chair with your feet about shoulder-width apart. The chair serves as a guide, providing safety and support during the exercise. Lower your body by bending at the hips and knees, keeping your chest upright and your weight centered over your heels. Imagine sitting down on the edge of the chair, but just before you fully sit, pause and then press through your heels to return to a standing position. This controlled movement engages the quadriceps (the muscles in the front of the thighs) and the glutes (the muscles in the buttocks), helping to build strength and endurance in these key areas.

Chair squats offer numerous benefits for seniors beyond muscle strengthening. By improving the strength of the quads and glutes, this exercise enhances the ability to perform everyday activities, such as climbing stairs, getting out of bed, or rising from a seated position. Stronger glutes also contribute to better posture and alignment, reducing strain on the lower back and promoting more efficient movement patterns. For seniors with limited mobility, chair squats are an accessible starting point, as the chair provides a safety net to prevent falls.

One of the best features of chair squats is their adaptability. If standing unassisted is challenging, seniors can begin by fully sitting and then standing up from the chair as an initial progression. As strength improves, the movement can be modified to increase intensity, such as lowering only partially or pausing longer before standing. These adjustments allow individuals to progress at their own pace while continually challenging the muscles.

Regularly practicing chair squats builds strength and confidence, empowering seniors to maintain their independence and perform daily tasks more easily. This simple yet effective exercise underscores the idea that strength training doesn't have to be complex to deliver meaningful results.

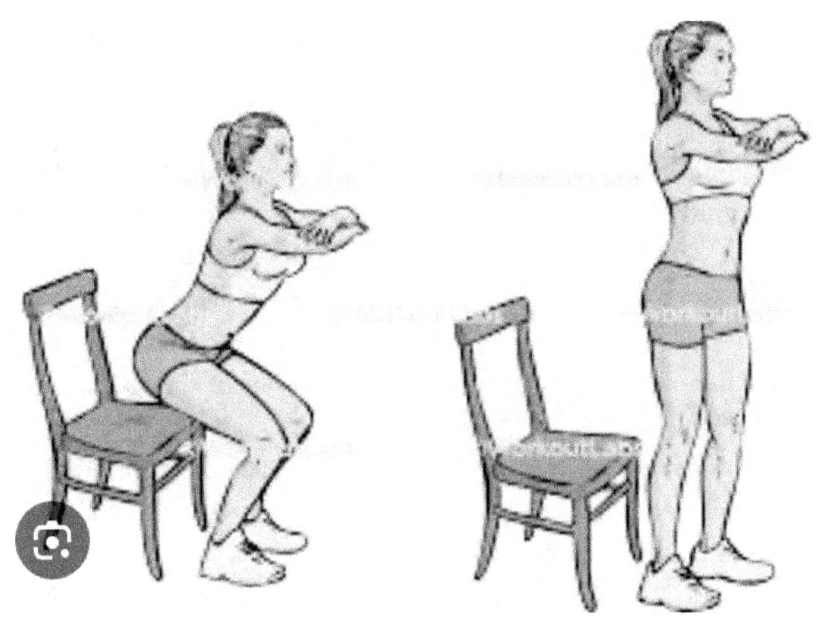

Calf raises for ankle and foot stability.

Calf raises are a simple but powerful exercise that targets the calf muscles, which play a vital role in ankle and foot stability. These muscles are essential for maintaining balance, walking smoothly, and supporting the overall structure of the lower leg. For seniors, calf raises provide a direct way to enhance mobility and reduce the risk of falls, which are often caused by weak lower leg muscles and instability in the feet and ankles.

To perform a calf raise, stand with your feet shoulder-width apart, holding onto a sturdy surface like a chair, countertop, or wall for balance. Slowly rise onto the balls of your feet, lifting your heels off the ground as high as possible while keeping your body aligned. Pause briefly at the top of the movement, then lower your heels back down to the floor in a controlled manner. This exercise strengthens the gastrocnemius and soleus muscles in the calves, which are crucial for stabilizing the ankle joint and generating push-off power during walking or climbing stairs.

The benefits of calf raises extend beyond muscle strengthening. Regular practice improves proprioception, which is the body's sense of position and movement. This heightened awareness helps seniors react more quickly to changes in surface terrain or unexpected shifts in balance, reducing the likelihood of tripping or falling. Additionally, stronger calf muscles support the ankle joint, making it more resistant to sprains or injuries caused by uneven footing.

Calf raises also enhance circulation in the lower legs by promoting blood flow through the contraction and relaxation of the calf muscles. This is especially important for older adults who may experience reduced circulation due to decreased physical activity or conditions like peripheral artery disease. Improved circulation can help alleviate discomfort, reduce swelling, and support overall vascular health.

One of the most appealing aspects of calf raises is their accessibility. They require no special equipment and can be performed almost anywhere, making them ideal for seniors with limited endurance or mobility. For those who find standing difficult, seated calf raises are a great alternative, allowing the muscles to be engaged with minimal strain on the rest of the body.

Incorporating calf raises into a regular fitness routine strengthens the foundation of the lower body, leading to greater stability, improved balance, and enhanced confidence in movement. This seemingly small exercise offers significant benefits, empowering seniors to stay active and navigate their daily lives with greater ease and security.

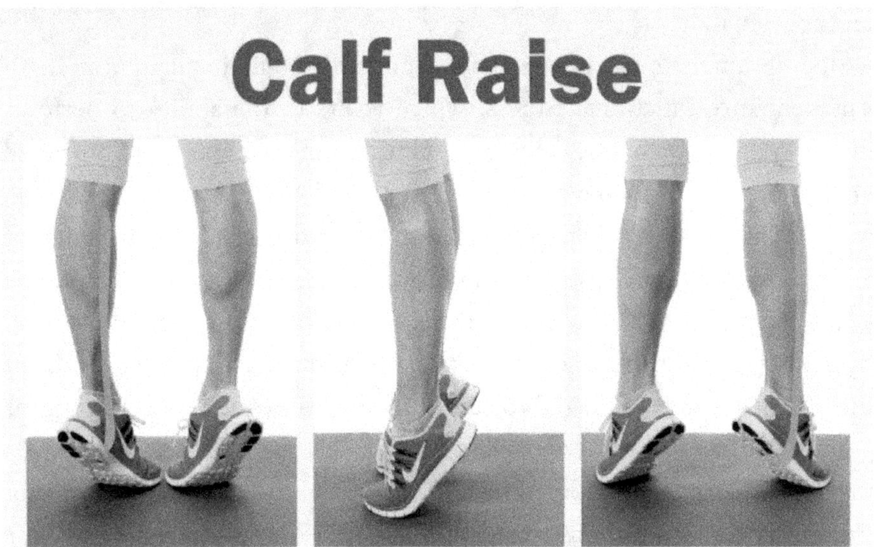

Step-ups for functional leg strength.

Step-ups are a highly functional exercise that strengthens the muscles of the legs while mimicking movements encountered in daily life. This exercise primarily targets the quadriceps, hamstrings, and glutes, while also engaging the calves and core muscles for stability. For seniors, step-ups are particularly valuable because they replicate actions like climbing stairs, stepping onto curbs, or getting in and out of vehicles—activities that require coordination, balance, and strength.

To perform a step-up, use a sturdy step, bench, or platform that is low enough to feel manageable but high enough to provide a challenge. Start by standing in front of the platform with your feet shoulder-width apart. Place one foot securely on the platform and push through that foot to lift your body up, bringing the other foot to meet it. Step back down carefully, leading with the same foot, and then alternate legs. This controlled motion strengthens the major muscle groups in the legs while also improving balance and coordination.

Step-ups offer a range of benefits that go beyond building muscle strength. They enhance functional fitness, which refers to the ability to perform everyday tasks with ease. By practicing the movement in a controlled environment, seniors develop the strength and confidence to tackle real-world scenarios, such as navigating uneven terrain or ascending stairs without assistance. Additionally, step-ups improve joint stability, particularly in the knees and hips, which are common areas of weakness for older adults.

Another key advantage of step-ups is their adaptability. The height of the platform can be adjusted to suit individual fitness levels, allowing for gradual progression as strength and confidence improve. For added safety, the exercise can be performed near a wall or rail for support, minimizing the risk of imbalance. Over time, variations like adding light weights or increasing the step height can provide an additional challenge, helping to further build strength and endurance.

Step-ups also contribute to better cardiovascular health, as the repetitive motion raises the heart rate and promotes blood flow. This makes them a low-impact way to combine strength training with aerobic exercise, providing dual benefits for overall fitness.

By regularly incorporating step-ups into a fitness routine, seniors can enhance their functional strength, balance, and coordination. These improvements translate into greater independence and confidence, enabling them to navigate their daily environments with ease and reduce the risk of falls. Step-ups are a simple yet powerful exercise that underscores the importance of practical, goal-oriented training for older adults.

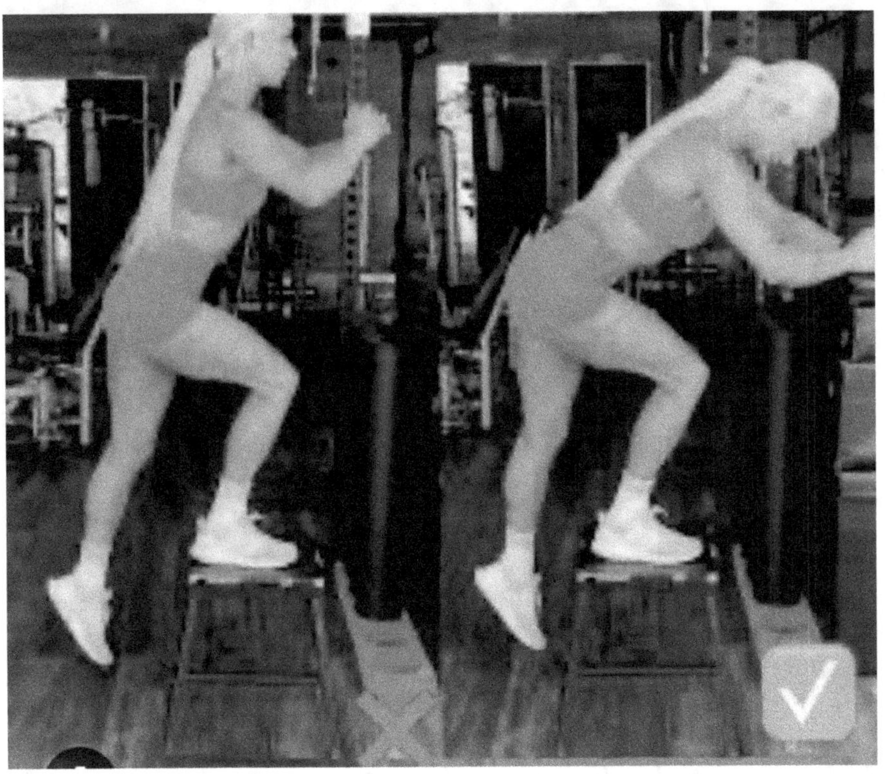

6

Chapter 5: Incorporating Resistance Bands for Added Strength

Getting Started with Resistance Bands

Resistance bands are one of the most versatile and accessible tools for strength training, especially for seniors looking to enhance their fitness safely and effectively. Getting started with resistance bands begins with understanding how to choose the right resistance level. These bands come in varying levels of tension, often color-coded to indicate the degree of resistance they provide. Selecting the right one is crucial; too little resistance won't challenge the muscles effectively, while too much can strain them. For beginners or those with limited endurance, starting with a light or medium band is usually best. Over time, as strength improves, progressing to bands with higher resistance levels allows for continued growth and muscle engagement.

Choosing the right resistance level.

Selecting the appropriate resistance level for your bands is crucial to maximizing the benefits of your workout while avoiding strain or injury. Resistance bands are typically categorized by levels of tension, often color-coded for convenience. Lighter bands provide less resistance and are ideal for beginners or individuals recovering from injuries, while medium and heavy bands offer greater tension for more advanced users or those looking to build significant strength. Understanding your current fitness level and goals is the first step in determining which band is right for you.

For those just starting with resistance training, choosing a band that feels challenging but manageable is key. When you stretch the band during an exercise, you should feel your muscles working, but not to the point of shaking, discomfort, or pain. If a band is too light, it won't provide enough challenge to stimulate muscle growth. Conversely, if a band is too heavy, you may sacrifice proper form, which can lead to strain or injury. A good rule of thumb is to start with a lighter band, master the movement, and gradually progress to higher resistance levels as your strength and confidence improve.

It's also helpful to choose a set of resistance bands that includes multiple levels of tension. This allows you to tailor the resistance to different exercises and muscle groups. For example, you may use a lighter band for smaller, weaker muscles like those in the shoulders and a heavier band for larger, stronger muscles like those in the legs. Having a variety of options ensures that you can target each area of the body effectively and progress at a pace that feels right for you.

Keep in mind that resistance levels vary slightly across brands, so the color-coding or tension rating may differ. Always refer to the manufacturer's guidelines and don't hesitate to test out a few bands to find the best fit. Remember, the goal is to challenge your muscles without compromising safety or technique. Over time, as you build strength and endurance, you can graduate to bands with higher resistance levels to continue making progress. Choosing the right resistance level is not just about the immediate workout—it's a step toward sustainable, long-term fitness success.

Learning basic safety tips for band use.

Using resistance bands safely is essential to ensure you get the most out of your workouts while minimizing the risk of injury. While resistance bands are a fantastic tool for strength training, their elastic nature requires extra attention to detail during use. Understanding and applying basic safety tips will help you build confidence and create a safe, effective fitness routine.

The first step is to inspect your resistance bands before every workout. Over time, bands can develop wear and tear, such as small tears, cracks, or fraying, especially if they are used frequently or exposed to heat and sunlight. Using a damaged band increases the risk of it snapping during an exercise, which can cause sudden and painful accidents. Always examine the bands for signs of wear, and replace them if they show any visible damage.

When using resistance bands, ensure they are anchored securely. If you're stepping on the band or wrapping it around a fixed object, double-check that it is stable and won't shift during the exercise. A slipping or poorly anchored band can snap back unexpectedly, leading to potential injuries. If you're looping the band around a piece of furniture or other structure, make sure the surface is smooth and won't cut or weaken the band material.

Maintaining proper posture and controlled movements is another key safety measure. Resistance bands provide continuous tension, which means it's easy to accidentally jerk or snap the band during an exercise. Instead, aim for slow, steady motions to maximize muscle engagement while minimizing strain. Avoid locking your joints, as this can increase pressure on them and lead to discomfort or injury. A slight bend in the knees or elbows during exercises can help protect your joints while maintaining control.

Safety also involves being mindful of your body's limits. Start with a resistance level that matches your fitness level and gradually progress as you build strength. Overexerting yourself by using a band that is too heavy can lead to poor form, muscle strain, or even injury. Listen to your body and stop immediately if you feel any sharp pain, dizziness, or discomfort during an exercise.

Lastly, create a clear and uncluttered workout area to minimize the risk of tripping or falling. Ensure there's enough space around you to move freely without bumping into furniture or objects. Wearing non-slip shoes and comfortable, breathable clothing can also improve your stability and overall workout experience.

By following these basic safety tips, you can use resistance bands confidently and effectively. Taking these precautions allows you to focus on building strength, improving mobility, and achieving your fitness goals without unnecessary setbacks.

How resistance bands enhance muscle engagement.

Resistance bands are uniquely effective tools for enhancing muscle engagement, offering benefits that traditional weights and machines often cannot replicate. Unlike fixed-weight equipment, resistance bands create variable resistance throughout the entire range of motion in an exercise. This means that as you stretch the band, the tension increases, requiring your muscles to work harder the farther you go. This continuous tension activates more muscle fibers, resulting in a deeper, more comprehensive workout.

One of the standout advantages of resistance bands is their ability to target both primary and stabilizing muscles. For example, when performing a bicep curl with a resistance band, not only does the bicep work to lift the band, but smaller stabilizing muscles in your arm and shoulder are activated to control the movement and maintain balance. This dual engagement helps build functional strength, which is particularly important for seniors looking to improve mobility and perform daily tasks with ease.

Another way resistance bands enhance muscle engagement is by accommodating your natural movement patterns. Unlike machines that often restrict your range of motion, resistance bands allow for greater freedom and flexibility, letting you perform exercises in a way that feels natural to your body. This adaptability helps ensure that muscles are engaged in a balanced and effective way, reducing the risk of imbalances or overuse injuries. For seniors, this is crucial for maintaining joint health and preventing strain.

Resistance bands are also incredibly versatile, making it easy to adjust the intensity of your workout. By simply shortening or lengthening the band, or by switching to a band with a different resistance level, you can modify the challenge to suit your fitness level. This scalability ensures that muscles are always engaged at an appropriate level, whether you're a beginner or more advanced. The gradual progression in tension keeps your muscles engaged and growing stronger over time.

Finally, the portability and flexibility of resistance bands make them an excellent option for engaging muscles in varied, functional movements. You can use them to mimic real-life motions, like pushing, pulling, or twisting, which helps strengthen the muscles you use most in everyday activities. This type of functional training not only enhances muscle engagement but also improves overall coordination, balance, and stability, key factors for maintaining independence and preventing falls.

In essence, resistance bands provide a dynamic and efficient way to engage muscles, offering a full-body workout that supports strength, flexibility, and endurance. They are particularly well-suited for seniors, as they are gentle on joints while still providing enough challenge to build and maintain muscle mass effectively. By incorporating resistance bands into your fitness routine, you can ensure that your muscles stay active, responsive, and ready for whatever life demands.

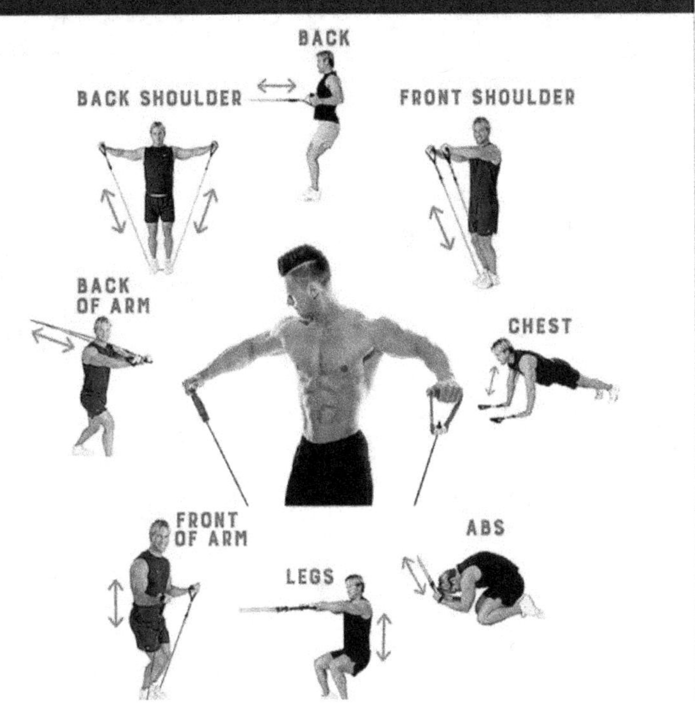
RESISTANCE BAND WORKOUT
FOR SENIORS
50 Resistance Band Exercises for Strength Training and Mobility
BACK
BACK SHOULDER
FRONT SHOULDER
BACK OF ARM
CHEST
FRONT OF ARM
LEGS
ABS

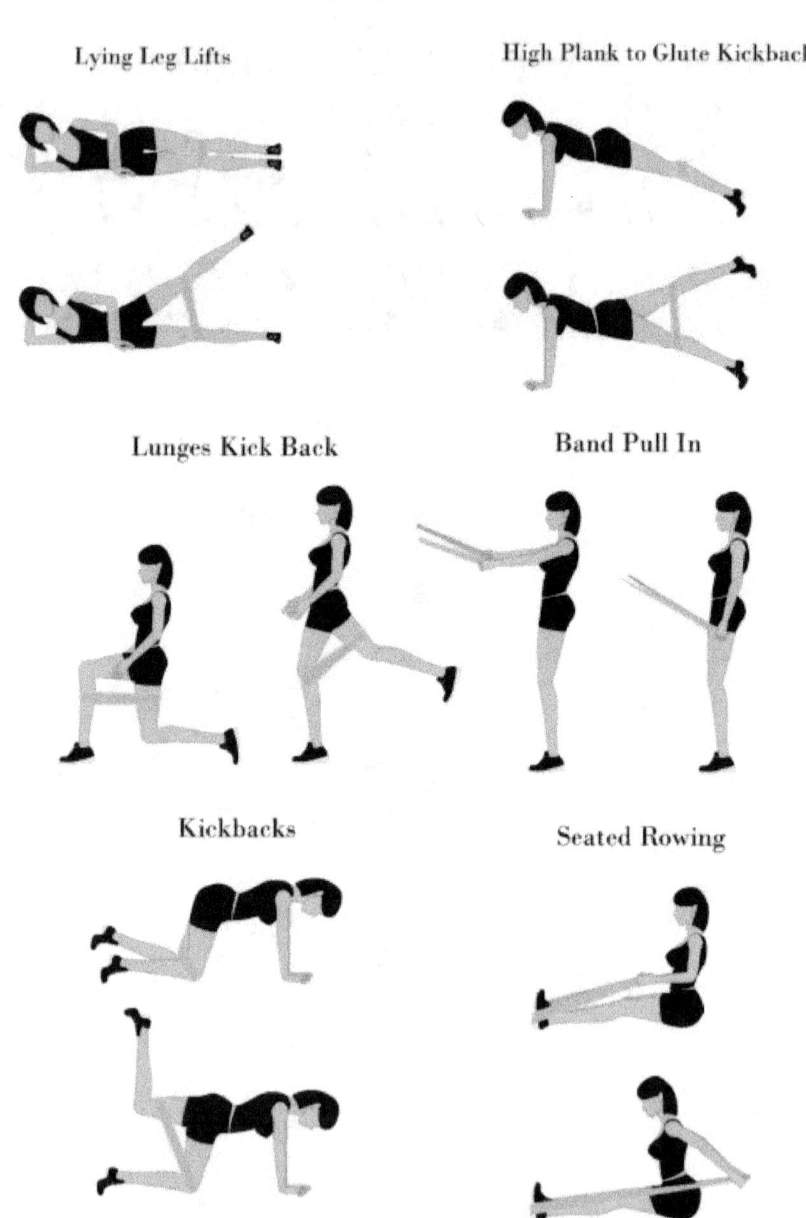

Lying Leg Lifts
High Plank to Glute Kickback
Lunges Kick Back
Band Pull In
Kickbacks
Seated Rowing

Upper Body Workouts

Building upper body strength is an essential component of maintaining independence and mobility as we age. A strong upper body supports everyday tasks such as lifting objects, opening jars, and even maintaining good posture while walking or sitting. This workout focuses on exercises specifically designed to enhance arm strength, shoulder mobility, and back stability—all crucial for functional fitness in older adults.

Bicep curls with bands for arm strength.

Bicep curls with resistance bands are a simple yet highly effective exercise for building arm strength, particularly targeting the biceps—the muscles on the front of your upper arm. These muscles play a vital role in everyday movements, such as lifting, carrying, or pulling, making them essential for functional fitness and maintaining independence as we age.

When performing a bicep curl with a resistance band, you start by anchoring the band under your feet and holding the ends in your hands. As you curl your hands toward your shoulders, the band creates resistance, which forces the biceps to contract and work harder. This resistance increases throughout the motion as the band stretches, ensuring that your muscles are engaged at every point in the exercise. Unlike lifting free weights, which can sometimes have "dead zones" where the muscles aren't working as hard, resistance bands maintain tension throughout the entire range of motion.

This continuous tension provides a more comprehensive workout for the biceps and also activates stabilizing muscles in your forearms and shoulders. These stabilizers help control the movement and maintain proper alignment, reducing the risk of injury and enhancing the exercise's overall effectiveness. Additionally, using a resistance band allows for a smooth, controlled motion that minimizes joint strain, making it ideal for seniors who may have arthritis or other joint concerns.

Bicep curls with bands are also highly adaptable, allowing you to modify the intensity to match your current strength level. You can increase resistance by shortening the length of the band or using a band with a higher resistance rating. This scalability ensures that you can start with a manageable challenge and progress as your strength improves.

Incorporating bicep curls into your fitness routine can lead to noticeable improvements in arm strength, which translates to better performance in daily tasks. Whether you're lifting groceries, pushing a door open, or simply holding onto a railing for balance, strong biceps play a crucial role. Over time, this exercise not only enhances the strength and tone of your arms but also contributes to overall upper body functionality and resilience.

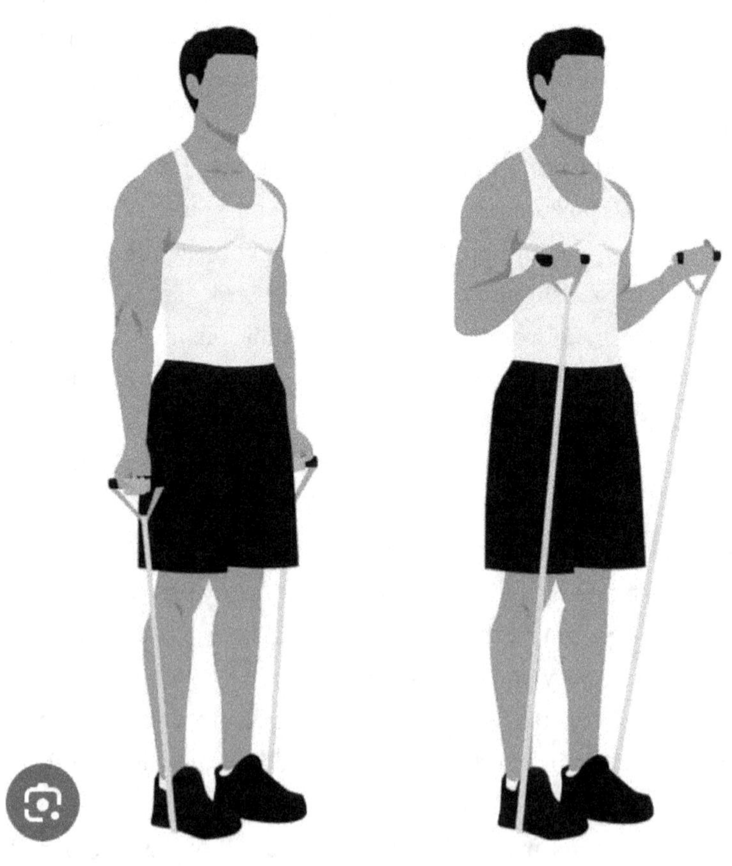

Overhead presses for shoulder and arm mobility.

Overhead presses are a foundational exercise that strengthens the shoulders and arms while significantly improving mobility and flexibility in the upper body. This exercise targets the deltoid muscles in the shoulders, the triceps in the upper arms, and various stabilizing muscles in the upper back and core, making it a versatile and effective movement for older adults.

Performing an overhead press with resistance bands involves pressing the band upward from shoulder height to a fully extended position above your head. This motion mimics reaching or lifting tasks you perform in everyday life, such as placing an item on a high shelf or reaching up to adjust curtains. By practicing this movement, you not only strengthen your shoulders and arms but also enhance your ability to perform these functional tasks with greater ease and confidence.

The repetitive motion of pressing upward stretches and activates the shoulder joints, increasing their range of motion. This is especially important for seniors, as shoulder mobility tends to decline with age, often leading to stiffness or discomfort during overhead movements. The overhead press gently encourages joint flexibility while simultaneously strengthening the surrounding muscles, providing both support and stability to the shoulders. This balance of strength and mobility reduces the risk of injury and improves overall joint health.

Another significant benefit of overhead presses is their impact on posture. Many people, especially as they age, develop a tendency to slouch or round their shoulders, often due to muscle weakness or prolonged sitting. Overhead presses help counteract this by engaging the upper back muscles, encouraging an upright posture. Strengthening these muscles not only improves how you carry yourself but also reduces the likelihood of developing back or shoulder pain caused by poor alignment.

Using resistance bands for overhead presses adds an extra layer of safety and adaptability compared to free weights. Bands provide consistent tension throughout the movement and allow for a smoother, controlled motion, reducing stress on the joints. Additionally, the level of resistance can be adjusted by selecting a lighter or heavier band, making it easy to customize the exercise to your fitness level.

Incorporating overhead presses into your routine is an excellent way to build shoulder strength, increase arm mobility, and maintain functional independence. With consistent practice, you'll notice improved ease in performing daily activities that require reaching or lifting, alongside enhanced posture and joint health. This simple yet powerful exercise is a key step toward maintaining a strong, capable upper body at any age.

Seated rows for back and posture improvement.

Seated rows are a highly effective exercise for strengthening the muscles of the upper and mid-back, which play a crucial role in maintaining proper posture and overall spinal health. This exercise primarily targets the rhomboids, latissimus dorsi, and trapezius muscles, all of which are essential for supporting an upright posture and countering the effects of prolonged sitting or slouching.

To perform seated rows with a resistance band, you begin in a seated position, either on the floor with your legs extended or on a sturdy chair. The band is anchored securely around your feet or another fixed object, and you pull the ends of the band toward your torso, mimicking a rowing motion. This action engages the back muscles as you squeeze your shoulder blades together, helping to build strength and stability in the upper body.

One of the key benefits of seated rows is their ability to address and improve posture. As we age, it's common for the muscles in the back to weaken, leading to a rounded shoulder posture and a forward head position. These changes not only affect appearance but can also cause discomfort, pain, and reduced mobility. By strengthening the muscles responsible for pulling the shoulders back and stabilizing the spine, seated rows help realign the body and reduce these issues over time.

Additionally, this exercise enhances balance and core stability. While the primary focus is on the back muscles, seated rows also engage the muscles of the abdominals and lower back, which work together to maintain proper alignment during the movement. This full-body coordination improves your ability to perform daily activities, such as lifting, reaching, or carrying objects, without straining your back.

Seated rows are particularly beneficial for seniors because they are low-impact and can be easily adjusted to accommodate varying fitness levels. Resistance bands provide a safe and adaptable way to perform the exercise, as the level of difficulty can be modified by using bands with different resistance levels or adjusting your range of motion. This makes it accessible even for those who are new to strength training or have limited endurance.

Regularly incorporating seated rows into your workout routine can lead to noticeable improvements in back strength, posture, and overall functionality. Beyond the physical benefits, standing taller and moving more confidently can also have a positive impact on self-esteem and independence, helping you feel your best in everyday life.

Lower Body Workouts

Strengthening the lower body is crucial for maintaining mobility, balance, and independence, especially as we age. The muscles in the legs, hips, and glutes are responsible for supporting your body during activities like walking, climbing stairs, and standing from a seated position. By targeting these areas with carefully chosen exercises, you can build the strength and stability necessary to maintain an active and confident lifestyle.

Band-assisted squats are an excellent exercise for working the quadriceps, glutes, and hamstrings while providing support for the knees. Many older adults hesitate to perform squats due to concerns about knee discomfort or strain, but using a resistance band can alleviate these issues. By looping the band around a sturdy anchor and holding onto it as you squat, you create an additional layer of stability that helps guide your movement and reduce pressure on the knees. This allows you to focus on proper form while gradually building strength and confidence. Band-assisted squats are particularly beneficial for improving your ability to stand up from chairs or low surfaces, making them highly functional for everyday life.

Side leg raises are another essential exercise for lower body strength, focusing on the muscles around the hips and thighs. These muscles play a key role in maintaining balance and stability, which are often areas of concern for seniors. By lifting one leg out to the side while standing or lying down, you engage the hip abductors and surrounding stabilizers, helping to reduce the risk of falls and improving overall mobility. This simple movement not only strengthens the hips but also contributes to better alignment and posture, as a strong lower body provides a solid foundation for the entire skeletal structure.

Hamstring curls round out a comprehensive lower body workout by targeting the muscles at the back of the legs. These muscles are essential for activities like walking, climbing stairs, and maintaining stability during movement. Using a resistance band for hamstring curls adds an element of control and adaptability, allowing you to adjust the difficulty level as needed. This exercise can be performed while standing or lying down, making it accessible for individuals with varying levels of fitness or mobility. Strengthening the hamstrings also reduces the likelihood of muscle imbalances, which can lead to discomfort or injury over time.

Incorporating these lower body exercises into your routine ensures that you're not only building strength but also improving functional abilities that translate directly into daily activities. Whether it's standing up from a chair with ease, walking with greater confidence, or maintaining balance on uneven surfaces, a strong lower body helps you stay active and independent. With consistent practice, you'll notice significant improvements in your strength, mobility, and overall quality of life.

7

Chapter 6: Using Light Weights for Targeted Muscle Growth

Introduction to Light Weight Training

Starting with small weights is one of the most effective ways to ease into a strength training routine, especially for older adults or beginners. Light weight training offers numerous benefits, including improved muscle tone, enhanced joint flexibility, and better overall stability. By beginning with smaller weights, you can safely build strength while giving your body the time it needs to adapt to new movements and resistances. This approach reduces the risk of injury and ensures steady progress without overwhelming your muscles or joints. Light weight training is more than just an introduction to exercise; it is a foundational step toward building strength, confidence, and better physical health. By starting with manageable weights, avoiding overexertion, and practicing proper techniques, you set yourself up for a safe and effective journey into strength training.

Benefits of starting with small weights.

Beginning with small weights is an essential step in establishing a safe, sustainable, and effective strength training routine. For older adults or those new to exercise, small weights provide the ideal balance of challenge and manageability, allowing you to focus on proper form and technique without the risk of overloading your muscles or joints. This measured approach is particularly important for those with limited endurance or pre-existing physical conditions, as it minimizes the likelihood of strain or injury while still delivering the benefits of strength training.

One key advantage of starting small is the opportunity to build confidence. Many people feel intimidated when starting a new fitness journey, especially if they're surrounded by images of heavy lifting and high-intensity workouts. Small weights remove this pressure, offering an accessible way to ease into training while still making noticeable progress. As your strength and familiarity with the exercises grow, you'll feel empowered to gradually increase resistance without fear of pushing yourself too hard too soon.

Small weights also help improve muscle endurance and joint stability. By performing controlled repetitions with lighter loads, you allow your muscles and connective tissues to adapt to new movements in a gradual and safe manner. This adaptation not only strengthens the muscles but also enhances coordination and balance—critical benefits for maintaining mobility and preventing falls, especially in older adults.

Additionally, starting with smaller weights provides an opportunity to fine-tune your technique. Proper alignment and controlled motion are essential for maximizing results and avoiding injury. Using small weights gives you the chance to focus on executing each movement correctly, reinforcing good habits that will carry over when you're ready to take on heavier loads.

Ultimately, starting with small weights is not about limiting your potential but about building a solid foundation for long-term success. By prioritizing safety, confidence, and control, you set yourself up for a fitness journey that's both enjoyable and effective.

Avoiding strain and overexertion.

One of the most critical aspects of beginning a strength training journey, especially for older adults or those new to exercise, is avoiding strain and overexertion. When starting a fitness routine, it's tempting to push hard in the belief that more effort will yield faster results. However, this approach can lead to serious setbacks, including muscle strains, joint injuries, and burnout. By adopting a gradual and mindful approach, you can ensure steady progress without placing undue stress on your body.

Strain occurs when your muscles or connective tissues are pushed beyond their capacity, often as a result of improper form, excessive weight, or performing too many repetitions. This can lead to microtears in the muscles, inflammation, and discomfort that may hinder your ability to continue training. Starting with lighter weights and manageable repetitions allows your body to adapt gradually, strengthening your muscles and joints over time without overloading them.

Overexertion, on the other hand, goes beyond physical strain and can impact your overall well-being. It often results from training too intensely, failing to take adequate rest between sessions, or ignoring signals from your body, such as fatigue or soreness. Symptoms of overexertion include dizziness, shortness of breath, and extreme muscle fatigue, which can not only derail your progress but also pose serious health risks. Recognizing the importance of rest and recovery is essential to building strength safely and effectively.

A key strategy for avoiding strain and overexertion is listening to your body. Pay attention to how your muscles feel during and after a workout. Mild discomfort is a sign of growth, but sharp pain or excessive fatigue is a warning to stop and reassess. Proper warm-ups and cool-downs, along with stretching, are also vital in preventing strain by preparing your muscles for activity and aiding in recovery afterward.

By focusing on manageable weights, maintaining good form, and progressing at a pace that feels right for you, you'll avoid the pitfalls of strain and overexertion. This mindful approach ensures that your workouts remain enjoyable and effective, paving the way for sustainable, long-term fitness success.

Proper grip and handling techniques.

Mastering proper grip and handling techniques is a fundamental part of strength training, especially when starting with weights. The way you hold and control the weight not only determines the effectiveness of your workout but also plays a significant role in preventing injuries. A secure, well-aligned grip ensures that the focus remains on your muscles rather than placing undue stress on your joints, tendons, or connective tissues.

A proper grip begins with positioning your hand firmly around the weight. Whether you're using dumbbells, resistance bars, or kettlebells, ensure your fingers wrap securely around the handle with your thumb locking into place. This provides stability, preventing the weight from slipping or shifting during an exercise. A loose or imbalanced grip can lead to poor control, increasing the risk of strain or accidents.

Another critical aspect is wrist alignment. Your wrists should remain neutral—neither bent forward nor backward—throughout the movement. Misaligned wrists not only weaken your grip but can also place unnecessary strain on the small joints and tendons in the wrist area. Maintaining a straight wrist that aligns with your forearm ensures that the force from the weight is evenly distributed, allowing for more efficient and safer lifts.

Grip strength also comes into play. For those new to weight training, your grip may fatigue faster than the targeted muscles. This is common and improves over time as your hand and forearm strength develop. To support this process, incorporate grip-strengthening exercises such as squeezing a stress ball or using hand grippers. Avoid over-tightening your grip, as this can create tension in your forearms and reduce fluidity during your workout.

Proper handling extends beyond just gripping the weight—it involves maintaining control throughout the exercise. When lifting, lowering, or transitioning weights, always use smooth, controlled movements. Jerking or dropping weights can not only disrupt your form but also lead to muscle strain or injury. Practicing mindfulness during handling ensures you stay focused on your technique, keeping your body safe and aligned.

By focusing on proper grip and handling techniques, you maximize the benefits of light weight training while significantly reducing the risk of injury. This attention to detail builds a solid foundation for more advanced exercises and ensures that every movement is both safe and effective.

Upper Body Weight Exercises

Building upper body strength with light weights is an effective and accessible way to improve your overall fitness and maintain mobility as you age. This section focuses on exercises that target key areas of your upper body, including the chest, shoulders, and forearms, ensuring a balanced and comprehensive workout routine.

Dumbbell chest presses for upper strength.

The dumbbell chest press is a foundational exercise that strengthens the chest, shoulders, and triceps while also engaging stabilizing muscles in the upper body. For seniors, this exercise offers a practical way to build upper body strength, which is essential for daily activities like pushing open doors, lifting objects, or even getting out of bed. The beauty of the dumbbell chest press lies in its simplicity and adaptability, making it suitable for individuals with varying fitness levels.

To perform a dumbbell chest press, you typically start by lying on a flat surface, such as a sturdy bench or even your bed if getting to the floor is challenging. With a dumbbell in each hand, you push the weights upward from your chest, fully extending your arms, and then slowly lower them back down. This movement primarily targets the pectoral muscles (chest), but it also works the deltoids (shoulders) and triceps (the back of the arms), creating a well-rounded upper body workout.

For seniors, the dumbbell chest press is particularly valuable because it helps counteract the natural muscle loss that occurs with aging, known as sarcopenia. Maintaining or building chest and shoulder strength improves your ability to perform everyday tasks more efficiently and reduces the risk of injuries from overexertion. Additionally, the movement supports joint health by encouraging a full range of motion in the shoulders, which can help alleviate stiffness and improve flexibility over time.

Using dumbbells instead of a barbell offers a distinct advantage, especially for older adults. Dumbbells allow each arm to move independently, which can help correct muscle imbalances and reduce strain on the joints. They also provide greater control over the range of motion, making it easier to modify the exercise to suit individual capabilities. For example, lighter weights can be used to start, with gradual increases as strength and confidence improve.

Beyond physical strength, the dumbbell chest press can also contribute to improved posture. Strengthening the chest and shoulders helps counteract the rounded posture that often develops from prolonged sitting or weakened upper body muscles. By incorporating this exercise into your fitness routine, you support a more upright and confident stance.

Safety is a key consideration, especially for seniors. It's important to use appropriate weights that feel manageable and to perform the exercise with controlled movements to minimize the risk of strain or injury. Starting with a qualified fitness instructor or physical therapist can ensure proper form and technique, helping you get the most out of this effective exercise.

Regularly practicing dumbbell chest presses can lead to noticeable improvements in upper body strength, endurance, and functional ability. Whether it's carrying groceries, lifting grandchildren, or simply feeling more self-assured in your movements, the benefits extend far beyond the workout itself. This simple yet powerful exercise is a cornerstone of any well-rounded strength training program for seniors.

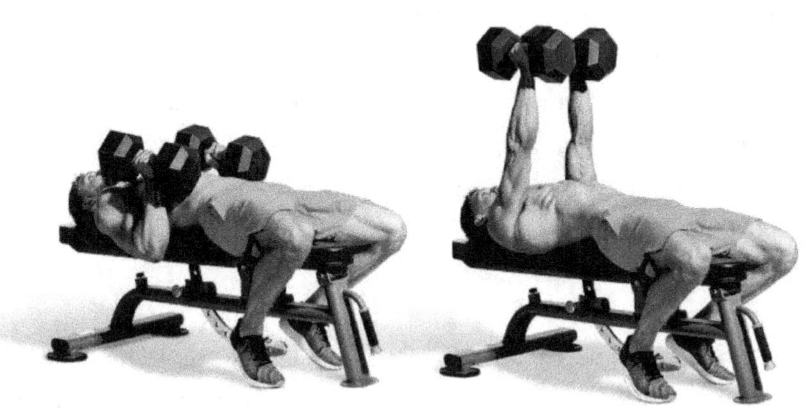

Lateral raises for shoulder definition.

Lateral raises are an effective exercise for targeting the deltoid muscles, particularly the lateral or middle portion of the shoulders. This movement not only helps build strength but also enhances the shape and definition of the shoulders, contributing to better posture and functional upper body strength. For seniors, this exercise is invaluable in maintaining mobility, improving stability, and preserving the ability to perform daily tasks with ease.

The exercise involves holding a dumbbell or resistance band in each hand, starting with your arms at your sides. From this position, you lift your arms out to the sides until they reach shoulder height, then lower them back down in a controlled manner. The key is to maintain straight arms (with a slight bend at the elbow to avoid locking the joint) and a slow, deliberate motion. This isolates the deltoid muscles and ensures they are doing the majority of the work, rather than relying on momentum or other muscle groups.

For seniors, lateral raises are particularly beneficial for improving shoulder stability and strength, which are critical for performing overhead or lateral movements in daily life. Simple actions like reaching for a high shelf, pulling open a door, or even stabilizing yourself when carrying items can become easier and more comfortable with stronger shoulders. Additionally, strengthening the shoulder muscles helps protect the joint from injury, which is especially important as joint resilience decreases with age.

Another advantage of lateral raises is their ability to enhance posture. Weak shoulders can contribute to rounded or hunched shoulders, which may lead to discomfort and a less confident appearance. By strengthening the deltoids, you support the upper back and encourage a more upright, balanced posture, reducing the strain on the neck and spine.

For seniors with limited endurance or mobility, lateral raises can be modified for comfort and safety. Using lighter weights or resistance bands is an excellent way to reduce strain while still providing an effective workout. Performing the exercise seated, rather than standing, can add additional support and stability, making it easier for those with balance concerns.

Consistency with lateral raises can yield noticeable improvements in shoulder strength and definition over time. This not only boosts physical capabilities but also enhances self-confidence, knowing that you are maintaining or even improving your upper body fitness.

It's important to pay attention to proper form to maximize the benefits and avoid potential strain. Movements should be smooth and controlled, and you should avoid raising the arms above shoulder level to protect the shoulder joint. Consulting with a fitness professional or physical therapist when starting can help ensure you're performing the exercise safely and effectively.

Incorporating lateral raises into a regular fitness routine can significantly impact your overall upper body strength, mobility, and appearance. Whether it's carrying groceries, playing with grandchildren, or simply feeling more capable and confident in your movements, this simple yet powerful exercise is a key component of staying active and strong as you age.

Dumbbell Deltoid Lateral Raises

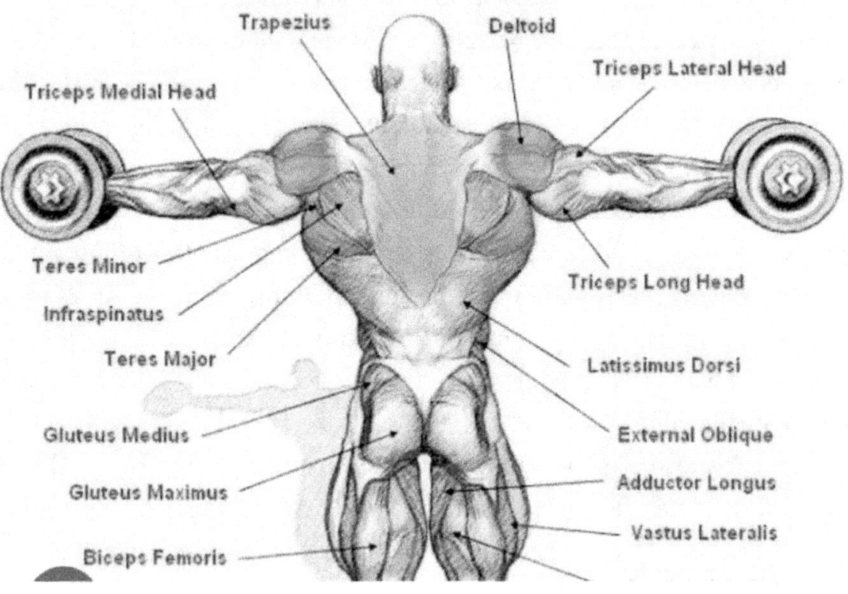

Wrist curls for forearm endurance.

Wrist curls are a foundational exercise designed to strengthen the forearm muscles, specifically targeting the flexor muscles on the underside of the forearm. This exercise is particularly beneficial for improving grip strength and endurance, which are critical for a wide range of daily activities, from carrying groceries to opening jars or simply maintaining a secure hold on objects. For seniors, who may experience a natural decline in grip strength due to aging or conditions like arthritis, wrist curls can help maintain or restore this essential ability.

To perform wrist curls, you typically use a light dumbbell or a resistance band. The exercise begins with sitting on a chair or bench, holding the weight in your hand with your forearm resting on your thigh or a flat surface, palm facing upward. Your wrist should hang slightly over the edge, allowing for a full range of motion. From this position, you slowly curl your wrist upward by flexing the forearm muscles, then lower it back down in a controlled manner. This movement isolates the flexors and ensures they are fully engaged.

One of the primary benefits of wrist curls is their ability to enhance forearm endurance. Many repetitive tasks, such as typing, gardening, or even leisure activities like playing a musical instrument, require sustained grip strength and stamina. By improving the endurance of these muscles, you can perform such tasks for longer periods without fatigue or discomfort.

For seniors, wrist curls are particularly valuable in preventing or mitigating conditions like carpal tunnel syndrome and tendinitis, which can result from weak or underused forearm muscles. Additionally, stronger forearms can help protect the wrists from injuries, as the muscles act as a stabilizing support system for the joint.

Wrist curls also play an important role in maintaining independence. Everyday activities like lifting a heavy pan, using a walking aid, or gripping the steering wheel while driving become safer and more manageable with strong forearms. This can have a profound impact on quality of life, allowing seniors to remain active and self-reliant.

For those new to exercise or with limited strength, wrist curls can be modified to suit individual needs. Starting with very light weights or resistance bands helps prevent strain while still providing a challenge to the muscles. Performing the exercise seated with a secure surface to rest the forearm ensures stability and reduces the risk of overexertion. Over time, as strength and endurance improve, resistance can be gradually increased to maintain progress.

It's important to maintain proper form during wrist curls to avoid unnecessary stress on the wrist joint. Movements should be slow and deliberate, with no jerking or bouncing. Keeping the rest of the arm stationary ensures the forearm muscles are doing the work, maximizing the exercise's effectiveness.

Incorporating wrist curls into a regular fitness routine can significantly enhance forearm strength, endurance, and overall function. For seniors, this translates to greater confidence in handling objects, reduced risk of wrist-related injuries, and an improved ability to enjoy the activities they love. This simple yet impactful exercise underscores the importance of addressing often-overlooked muscle groups in a comprehensive strength training program.

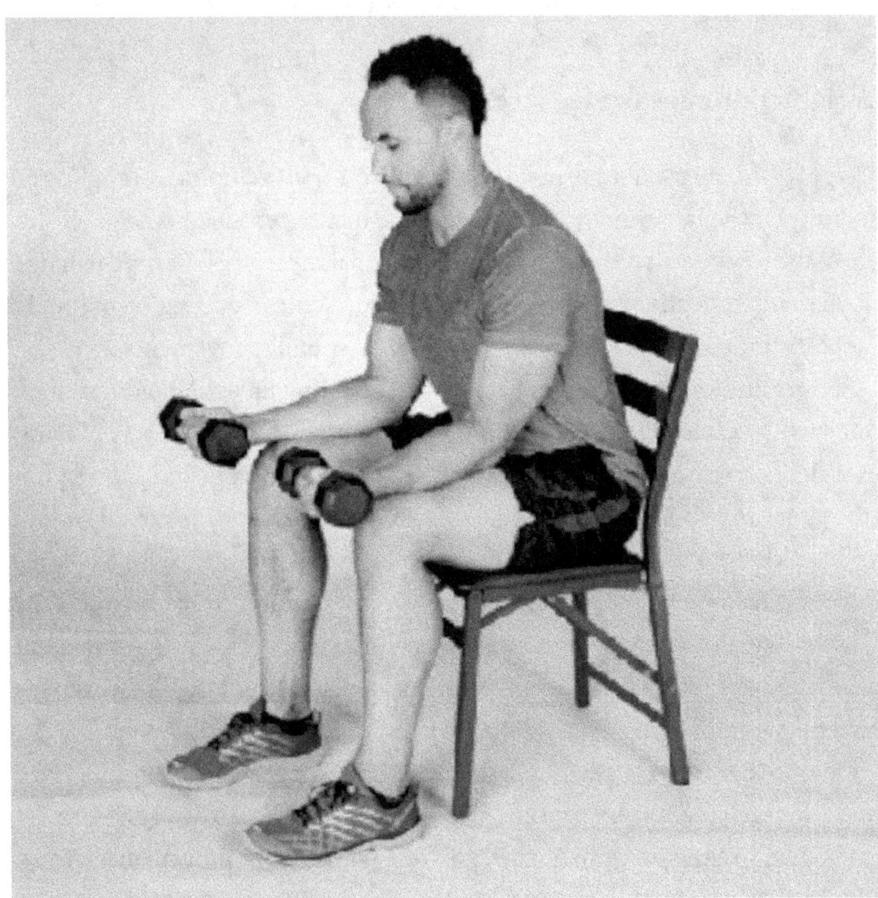

Lower Body Weight Exercises

Strengthening the lower body is crucial for maintaining mobility, balance, and independence as we age. Lower body exercises that incorporate weights add an extra level of resistance, helping to build muscle mass, improve bone density, and increase functional strength. This is especially important for seniors who want to stay active and reduce the risk of falls or injuries. Weighted exercises not only target the muscles of the legs but also engage stabilizing muscles in the core and hips, ensuring a well-rounded workout.

Weighted lunges for leg strength.

Weighted lunges are a cornerstone exercise for developing strength and stability in the lower body. They target the quadriceps, hamstrings, glutes, and calves, while also engaging the core for balance. This makes them one of the most effective functional exercises for seniors aiming to maintain mobility, independence, and confidence in their daily movements.

Performing weighted lunges begins with standing upright, holding a light dumbbell in each hand, or even using water bottles or other household items as weights. With a controlled step forward, you lower your body until your front knee forms a 90-degree angle, ensuring your knee stays directly above your ankle to prevent strain. The back leg bends slightly, with the knee hovering just above the ground. This movement not only strengthens the muscles but also stretches and activates stabilizing muscles, promoting joint health and flexibility. The weights add resistance, amplifying the workout's benefits without being overly taxing when properly scaled.

One of the greatest advantages of weighted lunges is their mimicry of real-life movements. Every time you bend down to tie your shoes, kneel to garden, or step up onto a curb, you're performing a movement pattern similar to a lunge. By strengthening the muscles involved in these actions, weighted lunges directly enhance your ability to carry out daily tasks with ease. This functional benefit is particularly valuable for older adults who wish to maintain independence and prevent injuries.

Beyond muscle strength, weighted lunges also contribute to improved balance and coordination. By requiring one leg to bear the brunt of the weight during each repetition, they train your body to stabilize itself. This is especially important for seniors, as balance can naturally decline with age, increasing the risk of falls. Regular practice of lunges helps counteract this decline, fostering better posture and control in movement.

To ensure safety, beginners can start with bodyweight lunges or lighter weights and progress as their confidence and strength grow. Supportive shoes, proper flooring, and a chair or wall nearby for stability can further enhance safety. Weighted lunges, when performed correctly and consistently, offer a practical and highly effective way to strengthen the legs, improve balance, and promote a healthier, more active lifestyle.

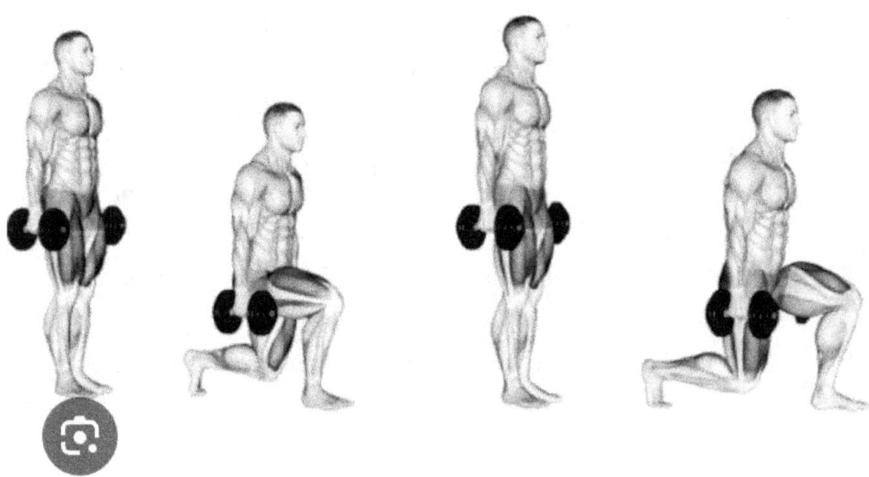

Heel lifts with light dumbbells.

Heel lifts, or calf raises, with light dumbbells are a simple yet powerful exercise that targets the calf muscles, enhances ankle stability, and improves overall lower body strength. This exercise is particularly beneficial for seniors as it promotes better balance, reduces the risk of falls, and supports the ability to perform daily tasks such as walking, climbing stairs, or standing for extended periods.

To perform heel lifts with light dumbbells, you begin by standing upright with your feet shoulder-width apart. Hold a light dumbbell in each hand, letting your arms hang naturally at your sides. Slowly rise onto the balls of your feet, lifting your heels off the ground as high as you comfortably can. Pause briefly at the top to feel the contraction in your calves, then lower your heels back down in a controlled manner. This slow and deliberate motion ensures the calves are fully engaged while minimizing strain or jerky movements.

Using light dumbbells adds resistance to the exercise, making it more challenging and effective. The additional weight helps to strengthen not only the calves but also engages stabilizing muscles in the feet, ankles, and core. These muscles play a crucial role in maintaining balance and posture, especially for older adults who may experience a natural decline in these areas due to age or reduced physical activity.

Heel lifts also improve circulation in the lower legs, which is important for seniors who may be prone to swelling or stiffness in this area. By encouraging blood flow and muscle activity, this exercise can alleviate discomfort and contribute to overall leg health.

For beginners or those with limited balance, performing heel lifts while holding onto a sturdy surface like a countertop or back of a chair can provide added stability. Gradually, as strength and confidence build, the exercise can be performed without support or with heavier dumbbells to further increase the challenge.

Incorporating heel lifts with light dumbbells into a regular fitness routine not only strengthens the lower legs but also enhances mobility, stability, and independence. This simple yet effective exercise can help seniors stay active and maintain their quality of life well into their later years.

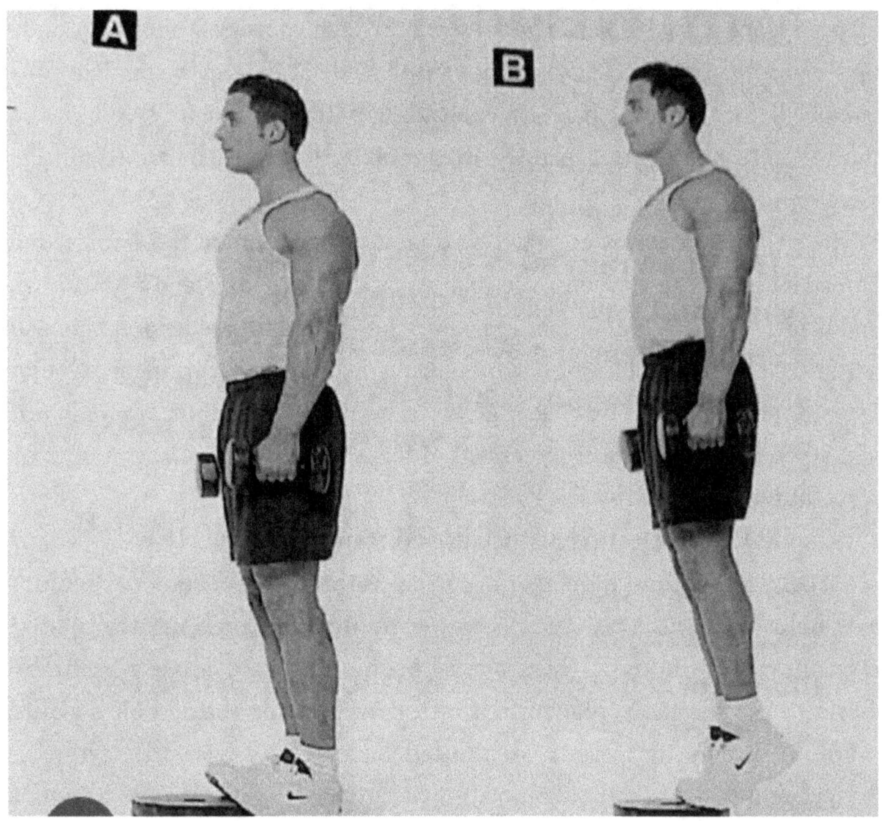

Weighted step-ups for balance and power.

Weighted step-ups are an excellent functional exercise for building lower body strength, enhancing balance, and developing power. This exercise mimics everyday movements like climbing stairs or stepping onto a curb, making it particularly valuable for seniors aiming to maintain independence and confidence in their mobility. The added resistance of weights increases the intensity, ensuring that the exercise strengthens muscles while improving coordination and stability.

To perform weighted step-ups, you need a stable platform, such as a sturdy step, bench, or low box, and a pair of light dumbbells. Stand upright with your feet hip-width apart, holding a dumbbell in each hand by your sides.

Step one foot onto the platform, pressing through your heel to lift your body upward until your other foot joins. Pause briefly at the top to stabilize your balance before stepping back down, leading with the same foot. Repeat the motion, alternating your lead leg after each set to ensure balanced muscle development.

The primary muscles engaged during step-ups include the quadriceps, hamstrings, and glutes. These are crucial for activities like standing, walking, and lifting. The calves and stabilizing muscles around the ankles and hips also play a key role in maintaining balance during the movement. By incorporating light weights, the exercise challenges your body further, helping to build not just strength but also power—essential for activities that require quick or forceful movements.

Weighted step-ups also enhance proprioception, or the body's ability to sense its position and movement. This is especially important for seniors as it helps reduce the risk of falls by improving reaction times and spatial awareness. Additionally, this exercise promotes cardiovascular health by elevating the heart rate, offering both strength-building and aerobic benefits.

For beginners or those with limited balance, it's wise to start with bodyweight step-ups or hold onto a sturdy surface for support. The height of the platform should also be adjusted to match your current fitness level, starting low and gradually increasing as your strength and confidence improve. Similarly, weights can begin light and be increased as the exercise becomes more comfortable.

Incorporating weighted step-ups into your fitness routine can make a significant difference in your ability to perform daily tasks with ease and confidence. This exercise not only strengthens the lower body but also boosts functional fitness, ensuring you stay active and independent as you age.

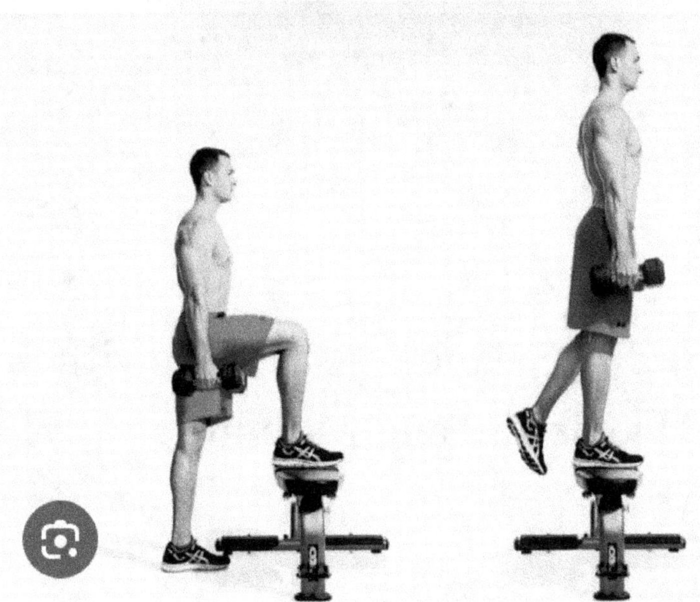

8

Chapter 7: Balancing Strength with Flexibility and Mobility

Why Flexibility Matters

Flexibility is one of the most essential yet often overlooked components of overall fitness, particularly for seniors. As we age, our muscles and joints naturally lose some of their elasticity, leading to stiffness, reduced mobility, and an increased risk of injury. By incorporating flexibility exercises into your routine, you can counteract these changes, keeping your body limber and improving your overall quality of life.

Incorporating flexibility exercises into your routine is not just about preventing stiffness or improving workout performance—it's about enhancing your ability to move through life with ease and comfort. Whether you're reaching for something, playing with grandchildren, or recovering after a walk, flexibility ensures that your body feels capable and resilient. It's a small investment of time with enormous rewards, allowing you to move more freely and enjoy your activities without limitations.

Preventing stiffness and improving range of motion.

As we age, stiffness in the muscles and joints can quietly creep in, making everyday movements less fluid and more uncomfortable. This stiffness is a natural part of aging, caused by the gradual shortening of muscles, a reduction in joint fluid, and a decline in collagen elasticity. Without intervention, these changes can lead to restricted movement and even chronic pain. However, by prioritizing flexibility exercises, it's possible to prevent or significantly slow this process, keeping your body agile and your movements smooth.

Preventing stiffness begins with keeping the muscles and connective tissues—like tendons and ligaments—active and pliable. Regular stretching encourages these tissues to maintain their elasticity, which is crucial for mobility. When you stretch a muscle, you not only lengthen it temporarily but also send a signal to the body to adapt over time. This adaptation helps the muscle and its surrounding structures resist the rigidity that comes with disuse or inactivity. The result is a body that moves with less resistance, making tasks like reaching, bending, and twisting much easier.

Improving your range of motion is equally important and is deeply tied to preventing stiffness. Range of motion refers to the full movement potential of a joint, from its flexion to its extension. Think of movements like lifting your arms above your head or rotating your shoulders—without regular stretching, these motions can become limited over time. Gentle, consistent stretches target the joints and the muscles surrounding them, allowing for more fluid and expansive movement. This enhanced range of motion not only improves your ability to perform exercises effectively but also makes daily activities—like putting on a jacket or stepping out of a car—much more manageable.

Another benefit of preventing stiffness and improving range of motion is the reduction in joint stress. When muscles are tight and inflexible, they can pull on joints and create imbalances, leading to discomfort or injury. Stretching alleviates this tension, ensuring that the load on your joints is distributed more evenly. For seniors, this can be especially crucial in avoiding joint pain and conditions like arthritis.

Incorporating even a few minutes of stretching into your daily routine can yield noticeable improvements in flexibility and comfort. Activities such as yoga, tai chi, or even basic static stretches can keep your muscles supple and your joints healthy. Over time, the consistent practice of stretching will not only prevent stiffness but also give you a newfound sense of freedom in your movements. It's a simple yet powerful way to maintain independence and continue enjoying life's activities without being held back by physical limitations.

Enhancing workout performance with stretching.

Stretching might seem like a simple addition to a workout routine, but it plays a transformative role in boosting your overall performance. Before diving into any strength training or cardio regimen, proper stretching serves as the critical bridge between your resting state and peak activity. It prepares your body to handle physical challenges more effectively while reducing the risk of injury.

One of the most immediate ways stretching enhances workout performance is by increasing blood flow to your muscles. When you stretch, you improve circulation, delivering oxygen and essential nutrients to the tissues that need them most during exercise. This preps your muscles for action, ensuring they are warm, pliable, and ready to contract efficiently. The result? You perform exercises with greater ease, precision, and power. For example, a well-stretched hamstring makes squats feel smoother, while limber shoulders allow for a better range of motion in overhead presses.

Another benefit is improved flexibility, which directly affects the range of motion in your joints. When you can move through a full range of motion without stiffness or restriction, every exercise becomes more effective. Take lunges or step-ups as an example: increased flexibility in your hips, knees, and ankles allows you to complete these movements with proper form, targeting the intended muscles more thoroughly. This not only maximizes the effectiveness of your workout but also ensures balanced muscle development.

Stretching also helps activate muscles that might otherwise remain dormant during a workout. Dynamic stretches—such as arm swings, leg kicks, or torso twists—wake up underused muscles, ensuring they are ready to contribute to the effort. By engaging these muscles early, you improve overall performance and prevent over-reliance on dominant muscle groups, which could lead to imbalances or injuries over time.

Post-workout stretching is just as crucial, as it aids in recovery and prepares your body for the next session. Stretching after exercise helps to release tension that builds up during physical activity, reducing soreness and stiffness. This allows you to return to your workouts sooner, feeling fresher and more capable of pushing yourself further. Additionally, stretching post-workout helps maintain the flexibility and mobility gains achieved during the session, making your progress more sustainable in the long run.

In short, stretching is not merely a warm-up or cooldown ritual—it's a performance enhancer. It improves muscle function, increases efficiency, and reduces the risk of setbacks caused by injury or strain. Whether you're lifting weights, walking, or doing resistance band exercises, incorporating stretching into your routine helps you move better, feel stronger, and achieve more with every workout.

Promoting relaxation and recovery.

Stretching is more than a physical exercise—it's a gateway to relaxation and a powerful tool for recovery. After a workout, your body needs time and support to transition from an active state back to rest, and stretching plays a critical role in this process. It helps release built-up tension in the muscles, calms the nervous system, and sets the stage for effective healing and regeneration.

When you engage in stretching after exercise, your muscles lengthen and relax. Physical activity often causes muscles to tighten as they work hard to stabilize your body and generate movement. This tension, if left unchecked, can lead to discomfort, stiffness, or even restricted movement. Stretching counteracts this by gently elongating the muscle fibers, restoring them to their optimal length, and relieving any tightness that may have developed during your workout. As the tension melts away, you experience a soothing sense of release that promotes both physical and mental relaxation.

Beyond addressing muscle tension, stretching triggers a calming effect on the nervous system. Deep, deliberate stretches encourage slow, mindful breathing, which helps activate the parasympathetic nervous system—the part of the body responsible for rest and recovery. This shift reduces stress hormones like cortisol and promotes a state of calmness, making stretching not only a physical relief but also a mental one. It's no surprise that many people find post-workout stretching to be as refreshing for the mind as it is for the body.

Stretching also facilitates improved circulation, which is vital for recovery. By increasing blood flow to the muscles, stretching delivers oxygen and nutrients needed for tissue repair while helping flush out waste products like lactic acid that accumulate during exercise. This accelerated delivery system aids in reducing soreness, preventing stiffness, and ensuring that your body is ready for the next activity sooner rather than later.

For seniors, this recovery process is particularly important. Aging muscles may take longer to recover, and stretching can help close that gap by optimizing the body's natural healing capabilities. Incorporating a stretching routine into your fitness program not only helps you feel better faster but also ensures you can maintain consistency without the setbacks of lingering soreness or fatigue.

Finally, the rhythmic and controlled nature of stretching offers an almost meditative quality, making it an excellent way to end a workout on a positive note. As you stretch, you're encouraged to focus on your breathing and the gentle movements of your body. This mindfulness can clear your mind, reduce stress, and leave you feeling rejuvenated and centered.

In essence, stretching isn't just about increasing flexibility or range of motion—it's about treating your body and mind to the care they need after exercise. By promoting relaxation and recovery, stretching ensures that you feel refreshed, resilient, and ready to keep pursuing your fitness goals.

Stretching Routines

Stretching is an integral part of any fitness program, and incorporating the right routines at the right times can make a significant difference in your workout performance and recovery. Whether you're preparing your body for activity, winding down after exercise, or simply looking to enhance your flexibility, stretching routines are essential tools to maintain and improve your overall physical well-being. Each type of stretching serves a unique purpose, and together they form a comprehensive routine that supports your fitness goals while honoring your body's needs. Whether you're preparing to exercise, recovering from a workout, or simply aiming to stay flexible and active, these routines ensure that you can move through life with greater ease, strength, and confidence.

Dynamic stretches for pre-workout preparation.

Dynamic stretches are a game-changer for anyone looking to prepare their body for physical activity, especially seniors. These stretches are active movements that gently take your muscles and joints through their full range of motion, mimicking the motions you'll use during your workout. Unlike static stretches, which involve holding a position, dynamic stretches keep you moving and help "wake up" your body for exercise.

The primary goal of dynamic stretching is to gradually increase your body temperature, heart rate, and blood circulation. This primes your muscles for action, making them more pliable and ready to handle the demands of exercise. For example, leg swings can prepare your hip flexors and hamstrings for movements like walking or squatting, while arm circles can loosen up your shoulders and chest for upper-body exercises. These types of stretches create a smooth transition from being at rest to engaging in physical activity, which is especially important for older adults who may have stiffer joints or less natural elasticity in their muscles.

Dynamic stretches also help improve coordination and balance, which are crucial for seniors aiming to maintain independence and avoid injuries. Movements like walking lunges or side steps challenge your stability and engage multiple muscle groups, creating a full-body activation that ensures your entire system is ready for activity. This not only reduces the risk of strains or pulls but also enhances your performance by allowing your muscles to function more efficiently.

Most importantly, dynamic stretching can significantly reduce the risk of injury. By preparing your muscles and joints for the specific actions you'll perform, you're minimizing the chance of sudden stress on unprepared tissues. For seniors, who may be more susceptible to injuries, this is a vital step in creating a safe and sustainable exercise routine. Dynamic stretches don't just physically prepare you—they also mentally signal that it's time to focus on your workout, helping you enter the activity with energy and confidence. Whether you're taking a brisk walk, doing resistance training, or engaging in yoga, dynamic stretching is the perfect first step toward a successful session.

Static stretches for post-workout cool-downs.

Static stretches are an essential part of any post-workout routine, offering your body the chance to transition smoothly from exercise to a state of rest. Unlike dynamic stretches, which involve continuous movement, static stretches are held in one position for a period of time—usually 15 to 30 seconds per stretch. This stationary approach targets specific muscles that have been engaged during your workout, helping them relax, lengthen, and recover.

After exercise, your muscles are warm and more pliable, making static stretching particularly effective. Holding a stretch encourages your muscles to release tension and return to their resting length, preventing the stiffness and tightness that can occur after physical activity. For instance, a seated forward fold can stretch your hamstrings after walking or leg exercises, while a standing chest opener can release tightness in your shoulders and upper back after upper-body strength training. These stretches not only feel good but also help reduce post-workout soreness, making your recovery process more comfortable.

Another critical benefit of static stretching is its role in improving flexibility over time. Consistently holding stretches allows the muscle fibers and connective tissues to adapt and extend their range of motion. This is especially valuable for seniors, as flexibility tends to decrease with age, leading to limited mobility and increased risk of injury. Static stretching helps counteract these effects by keeping your joints supple and your movements fluid, which are key to maintaining independence and overall quality of life.

Static stretches also promote relaxation, both physically and mentally. The act of holding a stretch encourages you to slow your breathing, focus inward, and calm your mind—a perfect way to wind down after the physical effort of exercise. This process activates the parasympathetic nervous system, reducing stress levels and fostering a sense of well-being. It's more than just a physical practice; it's a moment to center yourself, reflect on your progress, and appreciate the care you're giving to your body.

Incorporating static stretches into your cool-down routine is a simple yet impactful habit that supports your fitness journey. By improving flexibility, reducing soreness, and promoting relaxation, these stretches ensure your workouts end on a high note, leaving you feeling refreshed and ready to tackle whatever comes next.

Yoga-inspired moves for flexibility.

Yoga-inspired moves are a fantastic way to enhance flexibility, particularly for seniors, as they combine gentle stretching with mindful movement to improve both physical and mental well-being. Unlike standard stretches, yoga draws on centuries-old practices that focus not just on the body but also on breathing and relaxation, creating a holistic approach to flexibility training. These movements can be tailored to individual ability levels, making them accessible for older adults with limited endurance or mobility challenges.

One of the key benefits of yoga-inspired moves is their ability to target multiple muscle groups simultaneously while promoting balance and stability. For example, a modified downward dog can stretch the hamstrings, calves, shoulders, and back all at once. The cat-cow pose—a gentle flow between arching and rounding the back—helps improve spinal flexibility, loosens stiff joints, and increases blood flow to the muscles. These moves are particularly beneficial for combating the effects of aging, such as stiffness and reduced range of motion, by encouraging fluid, dynamic movement.

Yoga-inspired moves also emphasize proper alignment and posture, which are essential for maintaining joint health and preventing injuries. Movements like seated forward bends or gentle twists can stretch the lower back and obliques while reinforcing core strength, which is critical for supporting the spine and improving overall stability. The focus on controlled breathing during these poses also aids in relaxation and enhances the efficiency of your stretches, allowing muscles to release tension more effectively.

For seniors, another advantage of yoga-inspired moves is their adaptability. Many poses can be performed using props such as chairs, walls, or blocks to provide extra support. For instance, a chair-assisted warrior pose allows you to stretch and strengthen the hips and legs without compromising balance. These modifications make yoga accessible to individuals who may not feel comfortable performing traditional stretches on the floor or holding challenging poses for extended periods.

Beyond physical flexibility, yoga-inspired moves foster a sense of mindfulness and calm. Engaging in these movements encourages you to focus on your breath and the sensations in your body, helping to reduce stress and promote mental clarity. This mind-body connection is particularly valuable for seniors, as it supports emotional well-being alongside physical health.

Incorporating yoga-inspired moves into your fitness routine is an excellent way to maintain and improve flexibility while enjoying a practice that is both soothing and invigorating. These movements not only help your body feel more limber and capable but also provide a sense of accomplishment and tranquility, making them an enriching addition to your overall wellness journey.

Improving Mobility

Mobility is the foundation of an active, independent life, and improving it is especially crucial as we age. With the natural wear and tear that comes with time, our joints and muscles can become stiffer, making simple daily tasks feel like monumental challenges. However, the right exercises and approaches can help restore and even enhance your ability to move freely and comfortably.

Improving mobility is not just about physical benefits; it also has a profound impact on your confidence and independence. When you can move comfortably and without fear of stiffness or falls, you feel more in control of your body and your life. This empowerment motivates you to stay active and engaged, whether it's taking a walk, gardening, or playing with grandchildren. Mobility exercises remind you that age is just a number and that your body can still perform, adapt, and thrive with care and consistency.

Gentle joint exercises to reduce stiffness.

Joint stiffness can feel like an unavoidable side effect of aging, but gentle joint exercises can be transformative in maintaining comfort, range of motion, and mobility. As we age, the cartilage cushioning our joints can wear down, and the production of synovial fluid—our body's natural joint lubricant—tends to decrease. This combination can lead to stiffness, discomfort, and a reduced ability to move freely. Fortunately, gentle exercises can address these issues by keeping the joints supple and active, mitigating the effects of inactivity and aging.

Gentle joint exercises are specifically designed to promote movement without putting undue stress on the joints. For example, wrist rolls are an excellent way to relieve stiffness in the hands and wrists, especially for individuals who spend time gripping objects or typing. Similarly, ankle circles can help improve flexibility and circulation in the lower limbs, reducing swelling and stiffness after prolonged periods of sitting. These movements are low-impact, making them accessible even to those with conditions like arthritis or joint inflammation.

Consistency is key when it comes to reducing stiffness through joint exercises. When you regularly move your joints through their natural range of motion, you stimulate the production of synovial fluid. This fluid acts like oil in a machine, reducing friction and ensuring smoother movement. Additionally, gentle joint exercises help maintain the elasticity of the surrounding tendons and ligaments, which can tighten over time if left unused. By gently stretching these tissues, you prevent further restriction and discomfort.

Moreover, these exercises help to improve circulation to the joints. Better blood flow means more oxygen and nutrients are delivered to the joint tissues, which supports healing and reduces inflammation. For seniors, this improved circulation can also mean reduced pain and stiffness in problem areas like the knees, hips, and shoulders. Activities like shoulder rolls or neck tilts can ease tension that builds up from daily activities and improve posture, which often declines with age.

Gentle joint exercises are not just about physical benefits; they also encourage mindfulness and a connection with your body. Taking a few minutes each day to focus on these movements can become a form of self-care, helping you to feel in tune with your physical capabilities. They remind you that even small actions can lead to big improvements over time, giving you the confidence to move through life with greater ease and less discomfort. Whether you're starting your day or winding down, these exercises offer a simple, effective way to combat stiffness and maintain your independence.

Balance drills for stability and fall prevention.

Maintaining stability and preventing falls are critical aspects of staying active and independent as we age. Balance drills specifically target the muscles and proprioceptors (the sensory receptors in the muscles and joints that help us understand our body's position in space) that support stability and coordination. As we grow older, the risk of falls increases due to changes in vision, muscle strength, bone density, and reaction time. However, through targeted balance drills, seniors can significantly improve their stability and reduce the likelihood of falls.

Balance drills often involve exercises that challenge the body's ability to maintain an upright posture while moving or standing on one leg. For instance, standing on one leg—without holding onto a support—forces the muscles around the ankle, knee, and hip to engage to keep the body stable. This is an excellent exercise for improving proprioception, which declines with age and can lead to a higher risk of falls. Over time, consistent practice of these drills can help seniors regain their balance and feel more confident in their ability to navigate their daily environment safely.

Balance drills can be simple or more complex, depending on the individual's current level of stability. A basic exercise might involve standing on one foot while shifting weight from side to side. More advanced drills could include stepping over imaginary lines or using a balance beam or a low, stable step. These exercises help challenge the nervous system and stimulate the brain's coordination centers, encouraging better control over movement.

Moreover, these drills help in training the brain to respond quickly to changes in body position, whether due to an unexpected step or a minor trip. They promote quick reflexes, which are crucial for avoiding falls. By improving reaction time, seniors can react faster to obstacles and changes in their environment, potentially preventing accidents.

Balance exercises also engage the core muscles, which are essential for stability. A strong core supports the spine and helps maintain an upright posture, reducing the strain on the back and joints. Exercises like Tai Chi or yoga poses—both of which focus on balance, coordination, and breathing—are particularly effective for enhancing stability and flexibility. These activities not only improve balance but also contribute to overall well-being by reducing stress and promoting relaxation.

By incorporating balance drills into their routine, seniors can take a proactive approach to maintaining their stability and reducing the risk of falls. These exercises foster a greater sense of confidence in movement, allowing seniors to enjoy their daily activities with greater freedom and security.

Functional movements for everyday ease.

Functional movements are exercises that mimic everyday tasks and activities, making them incredibly valuable for seniors. These movements are designed to enhance the strength, coordination, and flexibility required for daily life, such as bending down to pick up groceries, reaching overhead for a high shelf, or stepping into and out of a car. By focusing on these practical, real-world movements, seniors can improve their quality of life, remain independent, and reduce the risk of injury.

Functional exercises often target multiple muscle groups at once, promoting a holistic approach to fitness that enhances overall strength and coordination. For instance, a squat not only strengthens the leg muscles but also engages the core and stabilizer muscles, which are vital for balance and posture. When seniors practice functional exercises, they improve their ability to perform activities they enjoy and need to do, whether it's gardening, walking the dog, or playing with grandchildren.

These exercises also help in developing the flexibility and range of motion needed to maintain an active lifestyle. For example, stretching exercises that involve reaching forward or to the side mimic the movements used in activities like gardening or driving. By improving flexibility and joint mobility, seniors can perform these tasks more easily and comfortably.

Functional movements also include exercises that train the body to react quickly and efficiently to unexpected changes in the environment. For example, an agility drill that requires seniors to step over obstacles or shift weight from one leg to the other can help them maintain their balance when they encounter uneven ground or obstacles in their path. This kind of training can prevent falls and injuries, allowing seniors to move confidently and comfortably through their daily routines.

Incorporating functional exercises into a fitness routine not only makes workouts more relevant and enjoyable but also contributes to better overall health. These exercises improve muscle endurance, which is essential for performing daily activities without fatigue. They also support cognitive function, as the brain works to coordinate movements and responses.

By focusing on functional movements, seniors can enjoy greater ease and comfort in their everyday lives. These exercises empower individuals to live independently, perform activities with greater ease, and stay active in their communities. They remind us that fitness is not just about looking good but about feeling capable and confident in the most fundamental aspects of life.

9

Chapter 8: Adapting Workouts for Limited Endurance

Recognizing Your Limits

Recognizing your limits is an essential part of maintaining a safe and effective fitness routine, especially as you age. It means listening to your body and being aware of when to modify exercises or take a break. Fatigue is a common indicator that you may need to adjust the intensity of your workout. It's important to identify the signs of fatigue—like feeling excessively winded, experiencing pain or discomfort, or noticing a decline in performance—and respond accordingly. This could mean reducing the weight, slowing down, or opting for a less intense version of an exercise.

Identifying fatigue and modifying intensity.

Identifying fatigue involves paying close attention to how your body responds during exercise. When you're feeling fatigued, it's important not to ignore the signs—whether it's heavy breathing, a rapid heart rate, dizziness, or muscle soreness that doesn't go away. These are red flags that indicate your body is under strain and needs a break or a reduction in intensity. It's not just about feeling tired; it's about recognizing when the tiredness is affecting your form, technique, or the quality of your workout. If you notice that your movements are becoming sloppy or you're struggling to complete reps properly, it's time to scale back.

Modifying intensity doesn't mean stopping altogether; it means adjusting your workout to make it more manageable. This could mean reducing the weight you're lifting, decreasing the number of repetitions, slowing down your pace, or switching to an exercise that is less physically demanding. The goal is to maintain a productive workout session without pushing your body beyond its limits. By making these adjustments, you can continue to challenge your muscles without risking injury or burnout. The key is to listen to your body's signals and be flexible with your workout plan, so you can build strength and endurance at a sustainable pace.

Understanding the role of endurance in fitness.

Endurance in fitness refers to your body's ability to sustain prolonged physical activity without feeling excessively fatigued or needing to take breaks. It's not just about being able to push through a tough workout, but also about maintaining a consistent level of energy throughout the day, whether you're running errands, playing with grandchildren, or simply walking around the house. As you age, endurance becomes even more important because it affects your quality of life and independence.

Endurance training helps improve cardiovascular health, strengthens muscles, and enhances the body's ability to use oxygen efficiently. This means that with increased endurance, you can engage in daily activities more easily and for longer periods without experiencing undue strain or exhaustion. It also contributes to better joint health and muscle tone, which are crucial for maintaining mobility and reducing the risk of injuries as you age.

To develop endurance, it's essential to gradually build up the intensity and duration of your workouts over time. This could involve activities like walking, cycling, swimming, or even dancing that elevate your heart rate and challenge your cardiovascular system. Understanding that endurance is not just about pushing yourself harder, but also about pacing yourself and allowing time for recovery, helps you create a balanced fitness routine that supports long-term health and vitality.

Balancing strength with cardio for overall health.

Balancing strength training with cardio exercises is key to achieving overall health and well-being, especially as you age. Strength training focuses on building muscle mass and improving muscle tone, which is vital for functional movements, balance, and preventing muscle loss due to sarcopenia. On the other hand, cardio exercises, such as walking, swimming, cycling, or even dancing, target cardiovascular health by improving heart and lung function, boosting endurance, and supporting weight management.

The synergy between strength training and cardio is what makes for a well-rounded fitness routine. Strength exercises build muscle and bone density, which not only helps with mobility and daily tasks but also supports metabolic health. Cardio exercises, when done regularly, enhance circulation, lower blood pressure, and improve insulin sensitivity, which are essential components of long-term health.

By combining both types of exercise, you create a balanced routine that enhances not just one aspect of fitness but multiple aspects. Strength training can boost your metabolism, making it easier to maintain a healthy weight, while cardio improves your stamina and overall cardiovascular function. This balanced approach helps you stay active, reduces the risk of chronic diseases, and supports a better quality of life as you age. It's about finding a rhythm that works for you—one that keeps your heart strong, your muscles toned, and your body resilient to the challenges of everyday living.

Low-Impact Alternatives

When traditional high-impact exercises aren't an option or just don't feel right for your body, low-impact alternatives offer effective ways to maintain strength, flexibility, and overall fitness. Chair-based strength training is one such option, providing a safe and stable environment for seniors to perform exercises that build muscle without putting excessive strain on the joints. Whether it's seated knee lifts, leg extensions, or gentle arm raises, these exercises allow you to work all major muscle groups without the risk of falls or excessive fatigue.

Chair-based strength training.

Chair-based strength training is a practical and effective way for seniors to build and maintain muscle strength, particularly when balance or mobility is a concern. This type of training uses a sturdy chair as the primary support, making it safer and more accessible for older adults. It offers an excellent opportunity to perform exercises that can strengthen major muscle groups without requiring you to stand or move around extensively.

When engaging in chair-based exercises, it's important to focus on exercises like seated knee lifts, leg extensions, or arm curls using resistance bands or light dumbbells. These movements are designed to build strength in the legs, arms, back, and core, which are crucial for everyday activities such as climbing stairs, carrying groceries, or getting out of a chair. By using a chair for stability, you can maintain proper form and minimize the risk of injury.

Moreover, chair-based exercises allow for progressive resistance training, where you can gradually increase the challenge by adjusting the weight of dumbbells or bands. This method not only helps build muscle strength but also enhances endurance and stamina, making daily activities easier and less tiring. Chair-based strength training is adaptable to individual fitness levels, making it a highly personalized way to stay active and achieve your fitness goals without the need for strenuous workouts.

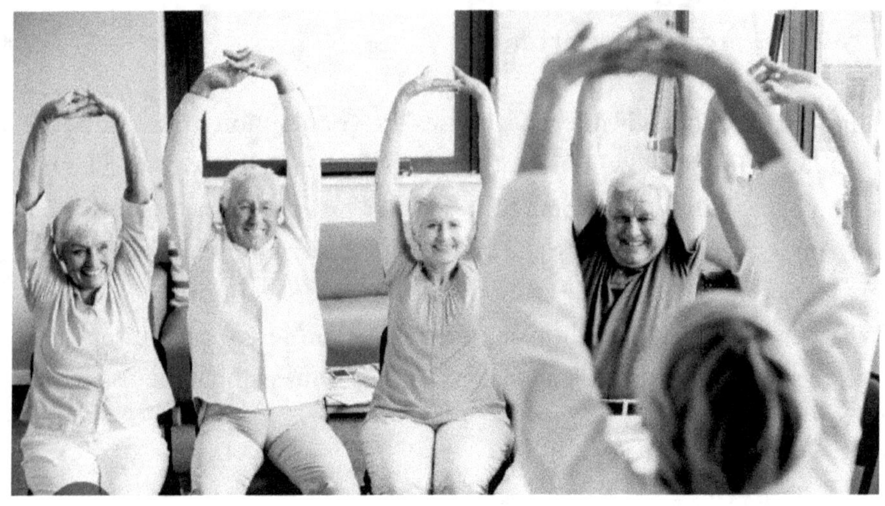

Pool exercises for joint relief.

Pool exercises provide an excellent low-impact workout that offers joint relief while still engaging muscles effectively. The buoyancy of water supports the body, reducing stress on joints, bones, and soft tissues, making it an ideal form of exercise for seniors dealing with arthritis, stiffness, or limited endurance. In the water, movements can be performed with reduced strain, allowing for a safer and more comfortable workout environment.

Exercises such as gentle walking, aqua aerobics, or resistance band exercises in a pool are designed to improve muscle strength, flexibility, and cardiovascular health without putting undue pressure on the joints. The resistance of the water adds a natural form of resistance that helps in muscle toning and endurance. This environment not only promotes joint relief but also enhances balance and coordination, crucial for preventing falls and maintaining independence.

Furthermore, the water's resistance can enhance muscle engagement and calorie burning, making pool exercises an efficient way to improve overall fitness. The buoyancy also supports better range of motion, which can aid in stretching and relieving tight muscles. Engaging in pool exercises regularly can improve mobility, reduce pain, and contribute to a more active and healthy lifestyle for seniors.

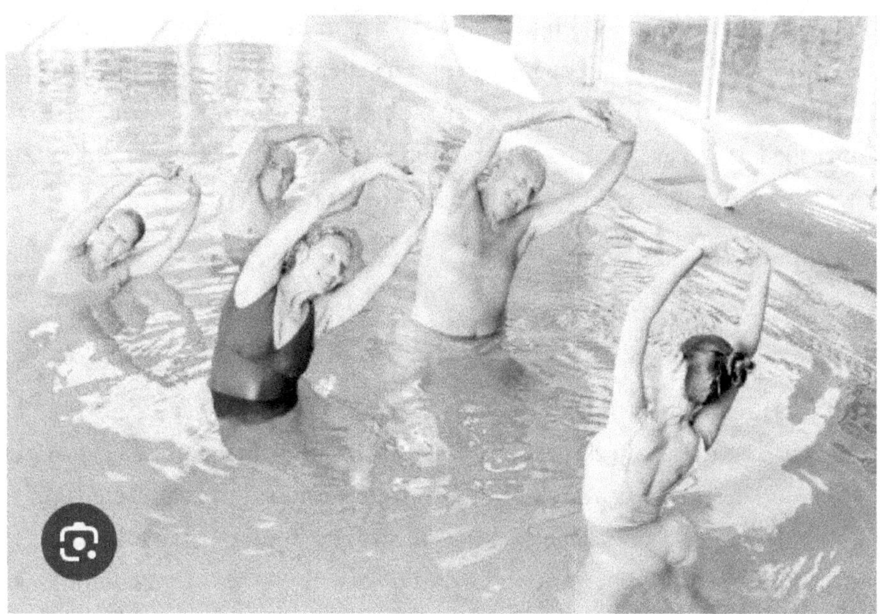

Slow, controlled movements for better engagement.

Slow, controlled movements are a key component of effective strength training for seniors. This approach emphasizes form, precision, and muscle engagement, ensuring that each exercise is performed correctly and safely. By moving at a deliberate pace, seniors can fully activate the targeted muscle groups, enhancing muscle strength, stability, and endurance.

These controlled movements help in developing better muscle memory and coordination. They allow seniors to focus on the muscle they are working on, making each repetition more effective. Whether it's lifting a dumbbell, performing a squat, or engaging in resistance band exercises, slowing down the movement ensures that the muscles work through their full range of motion, maximizing the benefits of the exercise.

Additionally, slow movements reduce the risk of injury by minimizing the chances of straining muscles or joints. This controlled approach helps in building a foundation of strength that is crucial for maintaining independence and avoiding falls. It also promotes better balance and posture, which are essential for overall health and quality of life as we age. By engaging in slow, controlled exercises, seniors can maintain a high level of fitness and enjoy improved physical health well into their later years.

Recovery and Rest

Rest days are not just a luxury but a necessity for seniors engaged in strength training. As we age, our bodies take longer to recover from physical activity, and adequate rest is crucial to prevent injury and support muscle repair. Taking a break from intense exercise allows the body to replenish energy stores, reduce inflammation, and rebuild muscle tissue. It's a time when the body repairs itself, adapting to the stress of the workout, and becoming stronger. For seniors, who may have more fragile joints and slower recovery rates, incorporating rest days into a fitness routine is especially important to avoid overuse injuries and burnout.

Importance of rest days for seniors.

Rest days are a cornerstone of any fitness program, but for seniors, they are especially critical. As the body ages, its ability to recover from physical stress slows down. Without proper rest, even light exercise can lead to overuse injuries, chronic fatigue, and setbacks in progress. Rest days provide the muscles, joints, and connective tissues with time to repair and rebuild, which is how strength is ultimately gained.

During exercise, tiny tears form in muscle fibers. Rest allows these fibers to heal and grow back stronger. For seniors, this recovery process is slower than for younger individuals, making rest periods even more essential.

Additionally, rest days help reduce inflammation that naturally occurs after physical activity, protecting against joint discomfort and stiffness, which are common concerns in older adults.

Rest days also support overall energy balance. Engaging in strength training or cardiovascular activities several times a week can be taxing on the body, especially if compounded by the daily tasks of life. By setting aside designated rest days, seniors can replenish their energy stores, ensuring they're ready for the next workout.

Beyond the physical benefits, rest days contribute to mental well-being. They give seniors a chance to reflect on their progress, recharge emotionally, and maintain motivation for their fitness journey. The balance between activity and rest ensures that exercise remains enjoyable and sustainable, rather than feeling like an overwhelming chore.

Using active recovery techniques like walking.

Active recovery is a gentle approach to rest that keeps the body moving without placing excessive strain on it. For seniors, walking is one of the best active recovery techniques. It's low-impact, easy to adapt to individual fitness levels, and provides multiple benefits for the body and mind without overloading tired muscles or joints.

When you engage in walking as an active recovery method, you're promoting blood flow to your muscles, which aids in delivering essential nutrients and oxygen to areas in need of repair. This enhanced circulation helps flush out lactic acid and other metabolic waste that can accumulate after strength training or more intense physical activity. The result? Reduced soreness and quicker recovery times.

Walking also keeps the joints mobile, preventing stiffness that might occur during full rest days. For seniors, maintaining joint flexibility is crucial for everyday functionality and avoiding discomfort. Gentle, rhythmic movements like walking ensure that the connective tissues stay lubricated and functional without the strain that comes with high-intensity exercises.

Mentally, walking can serve as a mood booster. A stroll through a park or around the neighborhood can be a relaxing way to connect with nature, clear your mind, or even catch up with friends. The light physical activity releases endorphins, which are natural mood enhancers, helping to reduce stress and maintain motivation for continuing your fitness journey.

Incorporating walking into your rest days doesn't mean you're pushing too hard; it's a way to strike a balance. It allows you to remain active, feel engaged, and support your body's recovery in a sustainable and enjoyable manner.

Monitoring progress and adjusting workouts.

Monitoring progress and adjusting workouts is an essential part of any fitness journey, particularly for seniors, as it ensures that exercise remains effective, safe, and aligned with individual goals. Keeping track of your progress allows you to celebrate achievements, identify areas needing improvement, and fine-tune your routine to better meet your body's changing needs.

Progress monitoring starts with recording baseline measures, such as the number of repetitions, resistance level, or the duration of exercises. As you continue, maintaining a simple log of your workouts can reveal patterns, showing where you've grown stronger or where you might be plateauing. This reflective practice isn't just about numbers; it's a motivational tool. When you see that last month you struggled to complete 10 chair squats, but now you're breezing through 15, it reinforces your commitment and encourages you to keep going.

Adjusting workouts based on your progress is equally critical. If exercises start to feel too easy, it's time to increase the challenge. This might mean adding more resistance with bands or weights, increasing repetitions, or extending the workout duration slightly. On the flip side, if you notice signs of overexertion—such as persistent fatigue, joint pain, or a prolonged recovery period—it's a cue to dial back the intensity or modify exercises to reduce strain. Your body's feedback is a valuable guide, signaling when to push and when to pause.

Flexibility in your routine ensures long-term success. Fitness isn't a one-size-fits-all endeavor, and what works one month might not work the next as your strength, endurance, and capabilities evolve. Tailoring your workouts as you progress not only keeps you engaged but also reduces the risk of injury by ensuring exercises remain suitable for your level. By regularly assessing how far you've come and making thoughtful adjustments, you're setting yourself up for continued improvement and a lifetime of health benefits.

10

Chapter 9: Staying Motivated and Overcoming Challenges

Tracking Your Progress

Tracking your progress is a powerful way to stay motivated and ensure steady improvement in your fitness journey. It transforms abstract goals into tangible achievements, allowing you to see exactly how far you've come. For seniors embarking on a strength training program, this practice not only fosters a sense of accomplishment but also provides insights into how to optimize your routine for continued success.

Journaling your workouts and milestones.

Journaling your workouts and milestones is an invaluable practice that turns your fitness journey into a measurable and meaningful experience. It's not just about recording numbers—it's about creating a personalized log that helps you stay organized, motivated, and reflective about your progress. For seniors, this habit can be a particularly empowering way to monitor improvements and maintain focus on long-term goals.

When you document your workouts, include details such as the exercises you performed, the number of sets and repetitions, the resistance level used (whether it's a band, dumbbell, or body weight), and how you felt during and after the session. Were the movements comfortable? Did you feel stronger or more flexible compared to previous sessions? Including such reflections helps you understand your body's responses and adapt your program to suit your needs.

Journaling also makes your progress tangible. Over time, you'll notice patterns: perhaps your endurance has increased, or you're lifting heavier weights with greater ease. These insights can be highly motivating, especially on days when progress feels slow. Looking back at earlier entries can remind you of how much you've achieved since starting your journey, providing a confidence boost when you need it most.

For milestone tracking, jot down specific achievements that stand out. Maybe you completed a full set of chair squats without support or managed a longer stretch of walking during active recovery. These moments of success are worth highlighting because they demonstrate tangible improvements in your strength, mobility, or endurance. Celebrating these milestones in your journal adds a layer of positivity and encouragement to your fitness routine.

Additionally, journaling provides a practical framework for troubleshooting challenges. If you notice recurring issues—like discomfort during certain exercises or slower progress in a specific area—you can use your records to pinpoint the causes and make adjustments. Sharing your journal with a fitness trainer or healthcare professional can also give them valuable insights into your progress and help them provide tailored guidance.

Ultimately, a workout journal becomes more than just a collection of notes— it's a roadmap of your fitness journey. It captures not only the physical aspects of your progress but also your mental and emotional growth. For seniors, this practice can bring clarity, confidence, and a sense of purpose to your strength training efforts.

Celebrating small wins along the way.

Celebrating small wins along the way is a vital practice that infuses joy and motivation into your fitness journey. These small victories may seem minor in the moment, but collectively, they represent significant progress and pave the way for larger achievements. For seniors, acknowledging and celebrating these milestones helps reinforce the idea that every step forward is meaningful, no matter how small it may appear.

Imagine the first time you complete a full set of chair squats without pausing or when you feel less winded after your daily walk. These moments reflect your hard work and dedication paying off. Celebrating them can be as simple as treating yourself to a relaxing activity, sharing your achievement with a loved one, or just taking a moment to reflect and feel proud. These acknowledgments help sustain your enthusiasm and keep you committed to your goals.

Small wins also serve as reminders of your capacity to grow and improve, especially on challenging days when progress feels slow. It's easy to become discouraged if you focus only on the end goal and forget to appreciate the progress you're making along the way. Celebrating small wins shifts your mindset to recognize that each step matters, creating a positive feedback loop that fuels further effort.

Beyond the psychological benefits, celebrating achievements helps build confidence in your abilities. If you were initially hesitant about trying strength training or doubted your capacity to improve, these small victories prove otherwise. They show that your efforts, no matter how modest they may seem, are yielding real, measurable results. This growing confidence makes it easier to tackle new challenges and push beyond previous limitations.

These celebrations don't have to be extravagant; they just need to be meaningful to you. Whether it's enjoying a favorite meal after a workout milestone, buying a new piece of fitness gear, or simply jotting the accomplishment in your journal with a proud note, these acts of recognition are powerful motivators. They remind you that fitness is a journey, and every step forward deserves acknowledgment.

By celebrating small wins, you make the process of strength training more rewarding and enjoyable. It becomes less about an abstract future goal and more about appreciating the positive changes you're experiencing right now. This perspective not only keeps you engaged but also makes the journey itself a source of pride and happiness.

Adjusting goals as you improve.

Adjusting goals as you improve is a natural and necessary part of any fitness journey, especially for seniors. Fitness is a dynamic process, and as you grow stronger, more flexible, or develop better endurance, your initial goals may no longer challenge or inspire you. Revisiting and refining your objectives ensures that your workouts remain effective, engaging, and aligned with your evolving capabilities.

When you first start, your goals might be simple: standing up from a chair without assistance, walking for ten minutes without discomfort, or performing a set of seated arm raises. These foundational targets are crucial for building confidence and establishing a routine. However, as you consistently work on these exercises, you'll notice improvements. That initial ten-minute walk may soon feel easy, or the chair exercises that once left your legs trembling might become effortless.

At this stage, it's time to reassess your goals. Instead of walking for ten minutes, you might aim for fifteen or twenty. Instead of chair exercises, you might progress to light bodyweight squats or incorporate resistance bands. Adjusting your goals helps you avoid stagnation and ensures that your workouts continue to stimulate progress. This process is called progressive overload—gradually increasing the challenge to your muscles to encourage further growth and strength.

Adjusting goals also keeps you mentally engaged. Sticking with the same routine for too long can lead to boredom or complacency. Setting new, exciting objectives reignites your motivation and gives you a fresh sense of purpose. For example, if you've mastered basic flexibility stretches, you might set a goal to touch your toes or improve your balance with single-leg exercises. These new challenges make your fitness journey feel dynamic and rewarding.

It's equally important to ensure that your updated goals remain realistic and achievable. While it's great to push your limits, overambitious targets can lead to frustration or even injury. For instance, if your goal is to increase the weight in your strength training routine, do so gradually, ensuring your body adapts without strain. Listening to your body and consulting with a fitness professional or healthcare provider can help you set safe and effective milestones.

This process of adjusting goals isn't just about physical improvements—it's about celebrating your growth and acknowledging how far you've come. Each new benchmark represents a step forward in your journey toward better health and vitality. Whether it's walking a greater distance, mastering a more challenging yoga pose, or lifting a heavier dumbbell, these new goals are a testament to your hard work and determination.

By regularly adjusting your goals, you ensure that your fitness routine evolves with you. It keeps your workouts challenging yet enjoyable, helping you maintain progress while avoiding plateaus. Most importantly, it fosters a mindset of lifelong improvement, reminding you that fitness is not a destination but a continuous journey of self-discovery and growth.

Dealing with Setbacks

Setbacks are an inevitable part of any fitness journey, and for seniors, they can sometimes feel more discouraging due to the physical and emotional challenges that come with aging. Whether it's an injury, a health issue, or a temporary lack of motivation, these moments can test your commitment. However, setbacks don't define your progress—how you respond to them does. Setbacks don't have to stop your progress; they can shape it. With patience, perspective, and the right support, you can turn obstacles into stepping stones on your path to a healthier, stronger, and more empowered you.

Managing injuries or health issues

.Managing injuries or health issues requires a thoughtful and proactive approach to ensure that you maintain your safety and continue progressing toward your fitness goals. Injuries and health challenges are common, especially as we age, but they don't have to derail your journey entirely. The key lies in addressing these issues promptly and responsibly.

When an injury occurs, the first step is to stop any activity that exacerbates the pain or discomfort. Pushing through an injury can worsen the condition and lead to long-term setbacks. Instead, seek professional advice from a doctor or physical therapist. These experts can assess the severity of the issue and recommend appropriate treatments, modifications, or rest periods. For chronic health conditions such as arthritis, diabetes, or heart issues, consult your healthcare provider before beginning or altering your exercise routine to ensure your activities align with your overall health needs.

Sometimes managing an injury or health problem means modifying your workouts. Low-impact exercises or alternative movements can help you stay active while avoiding strain on the affected area. For example, pool-based exercises might be a safer option if joint pain is a concern, or chair-based routines could allow you to maintain strength without exacerbating an injury. By adapting your routine, you remain consistent without putting undue pressure on your body.

Recovery is another essential aspect of managing health issues. Resting injured areas, following prescribed therapies, and gradually reintroducing exercises help your body heal and strengthen. Avoid the temptation to rush back into your full routine, as this can delay healing or increase the risk of re-injury. Instead, focus on incremental progress, celebrating each small step as a victory.

Finally, pay close attention to your body's signals. Fatigue, swelling, or prolonged pain are indicators that adjustments might be necessary. Learning to listen to these cues and respond appropriately is a vital skill that promotes long-term fitness and well-being. Managing injuries and health issues with care and patience ensures that these temporary challenges don't become permanent obstacles in your fitness journey.

Reframing negative thoughts into motivation.

Reframing negative thoughts into motivation is a powerful mental shift that can help you overcome challenges and maintain your commitment to fitness, even when setbacks arise. Negative thoughts often emerge from frustration, self-doubt, or comparisons to others, but by changing how you interpret these thoughts, you can use them to fuel your progress instead of holding you back.

When you encounter a setback or feel discouraged, it's natural to think things like, *"I'll never get better"* or *"I'm too old to keep up."* These thoughts, while understandable, can become self-fulfilling if left unchecked. Reframing involves recognizing these patterns and replacing them with empowering alternatives. For example, instead of thinking, *"I can't do this anymore,"* shift to, *"I'm facing a challenge, but I've overcome others before, and I can adapt again."* This reframing turns a defeatist mindset into one that is solution-oriented and resilient.

A helpful strategy for reframing is to focus on what you've already achieved. Reflect on your past successes, no matter how small they might seem. Perhaps you've gained strength, improved flexibility, or maintained consistency with your workouts. These accomplishments demonstrate your ability to persevere and can provide the confidence needed to face current obstacles. Remembering how far you've come can help you see setbacks as temporary hurdles rather than permanent roadblocks.

Another approach is to set small, immediate goals to redirect your focus. For instance, if you're feeling frustrated about an injury that limits your range of motion, set a goal to improve your flexibility in another area or practice mindfulness exercises. Shifting attention to what you *can* control keeps you moving forward and reduces the weight of negative emotions.

Gratitude can also play a significant role in reframing negativity. Instead of focusing on what you can't do, remind yourself of what you're still capable of achieving. Acknowledge your body's ability to heal, adapt, and grow stronger over time. This mindset fosters optimism and inspires you to work within your current abilities while looking forward to continued improvement.

Ultimately, reframing negative thoughts is about perspective. By choosing to view challenges as opportunities for growth and setbacks as temporary detours, you create a mental environment where motivation thrives. This mindset not only keeps you on track with your fitness goals but also strengthens your resilience in all aspects of life.

Creating a support network for encouragement.

Creating a support network for encouragement is an essential step in staying committed to your fitness journey, especially when challenges arise. A strong support network offers emotional reinforcement, practical advice, and a sense of accountability, making it easier to maintain motivation and overcome obstacles.

Your support network can include family, friends, fitness professionals, or like-minded individuals with similar goals. Sharing your fitness aspirations with those around you helps foster understanding and encouragement. For instance, letting your family know you're working on improving your strength can inspire them to cheer you on, celebrate your progress, or even join you in some activities. Their positive reinforcement can make a significant difference, especially during moments when your enthusiasm wanes.

Fitness groups or classes tailored to seniors can also provide a valuable sense of community. These environments allow you to connect with others who share similar experiences and challenges. The camaraderie in such settings not only builds friendships but also serves as a source of mutual motivation. Seeing others succeed, adapt, or persevere can inspire you to keep pushing forward.

In some cases, a fitness coach or physical therapist may be a key part of your support system. These professionals can provide expert guidance and personalized encouragement, helping you navigate your goals safely and effectively. They can also help you recognize progress that might not be immediately apparent, boosting your confidence along the way.

Online communities and social media groups focused on senior fitness are another excellent resource for creating a support network. These platforms allow you to exchange tips, share your journey, and receive encouragement from people all over the world. Being part of a virtual group can help you feel connected and supported, even if in-person options are limited.

Finally, don't overlook the importance of self-support. Encouraging yourself through positive self-talk, journaling achievements, or setting up small rewards for milestones can reinforce your motivation. Surrounding yourself with individuals who inspire and uplift you, both in real life and online, creates an ecosystem of encouragement that keeps you engaged and optimistic.

A strong support network helps you stay focused on your goals and provides a safety net during setbacks. It transforms fitness from a solitary effort into a collective journey, making the process more enjoyable, sustainable, and successful.

Maintaining Consistency

Maintaining consistency in your fitness routine is the cornerstone of achieving long-term results and reaping the many benefits of regular exercise. One of the most effective ways to stay consistent is by setting a regular workout schedule. Establishing specific days and times for exercise helps create a sense of routine and discipline, making workouts a non-negotiable part of your week. Whether it's a morning stretch session or an afternoon strength workout, a consistent schedule turns fitness into a natural and integral part of your lifestyle.

Setting a regular workout schedule.

Setting a regular workout schedule is an essential strategy for maintaining consistency and building a long-lasting fitness habit. A defined schedule helps create structure in your routine, making it easier to prioritize exercise even on busy days. When you dedicate specific times to your workouts, they become a natural and expected part of your daily or weekly rhythm, reducing the likelihood of skipping sessions due to lack of time or motivation.

To create an effective schedule, consider your personal preferences and energy levels throughout the day. For example, if you feel more energetic in the morning, plan your workout during that time to set a positive tone for the day. If afternoons or evenings work better for you, align your sessions with those periods when you can fully commit. Consistency in timing reinforces the habit, allowing your body and mind to anticipate and prepare for exercise.

Flexibility within your schedule is equally important to accommodate unexpected events or changes. While consistency is the goal, it's helpful to have backup options, such as shorter workouts or alternate days, to keep the momentum going when life gets busy. Remember that even a brief session contributes to your overall progress, so don't let small disruptions derail your commitment.

By viewing your workouts as a priority and carving out dedicated time for them, you're more likely to stay on track and make fitness an integral part of your life. Over time, this regularity helps reinforce the importance of exercise in maintaining your health and well-being, turning it into a habit that requires little extra effort to maintain.

Finding enjoyment in your routine.

Finding enjoyment in your routine is a critical factor in sustaining motivation and making fitness a long-term habit. When exercise is fun, it becomes something you look forward to rather than a chore. Enjoyment can come from a variety of sources, such as the type of activity you choose, the environment, or the people you engage with during your workouts.

To find joy in your fitness routine, start by exploring different types of activities to see what you truly enjoy. Whether it's dancing, cycling, swimming, yoga, or strength training, there's a wide range of options to suit various preferences and fitness levels. Experimenting with different exercises can help you discover what resonates with you and what you find most enjoyable. When you enjoy what you're doing, you're more likely to stick with it and make it a consistent part of your life.

Another way to enhance enjoyment is by incorporating variety into your routine. Doing the same exercises day after day can become monotonous and lead to burnout. Mixing up your workouts with different activities, classes, or routines keeps things fresh and exciting. You might find joy in trying a new fitness class, joining a local sports league, or going for a nature hike on weekends. Variety not only keeps you engaged but also challenges different muscle groups and helps prevent plateaus.

Socializing during workouts can also make fitness more enjoyable. Whether it's working out with a friend, joining a fitness group, or attending community events, social interactions can add a sense of camaraderie and motivation. Having someone to exercise with can make sessions more enjoyable and provide mutual support, accountability, and encouragement.

Ultimately, finding enjoyment in your routine is about connecting with activities that bring you joy and satisfaction. When you enjoy exercise, it becomes a positive and rewarding experience rather than a burdensome task, which makes it easier to stay consistent and committed to your fitness journey.

Keeping fitness a lifelong habit.

Keeping fitness a lifelong habit requires a combination of mindset, adaptability, and commitment. It's about viewing exercise not just as a temporary goal or a quick fix, but as an integral part of a healthy, balanced lifestyle that you sustain throughout the years. Achieving this means setting realistic expectations, staying flexible with your routine, and making exercise a priority in your daily life.

One of the keys to turning fitness into a lifelong habit is developing a strong, intrinsic motivation. Instead of focusing solely on external goals like weight loss or appearance, consider how regular physical activity can enhance your overall quality of life. This might include benefits like improved mental health, better energy levels, enhanced strength, and the ability to engage in daily activities with ease. When you connect exercise to these broader life benefits, you're more likely to stick with it even when faced with obstacles or challenges.

Adaptability is also crucial for maintaining a lifelong fitness habit. Life is constantly changing, and so too should your fitness routine. As you age or as circumstances in your life change, your exercise needs and preferences might evolve. This could mean trying new activities, modifying exercises to accommodate injuries or limitations, or adjusting the intensity to match your current fitness level. Being flexible allows you to adapt your fitness routine to continue challenging yourself and enjoying exercise, regardless of what else is going on in your life.

Incorporating fitness into your daily life in small, manageable ways can also help you maintain it as a lifelong habit. This could involve integrating physical activity into routine tasks like taking the stairs instead of the elevator, walking or cycling for errands, or standing up every hour to stretch and move. Making these small changes helps embed fitness into your daily routine and reduces the risk of it being neglected.

Finally, building a support system is vital for sustaining fitness as a lifelong habit. This could include friends, family members, or online communities who share similar fitness goals and can offer encouragement, accountability, and motivation. Having people to exercise with, share progress with, or simply chat about fitness can make the journey more enjoyable and increase your commitment to maintaining a healthy lifestyle over the long term.

By maintaining an adaptable mindset, finding intrinsic motivation, integrating physical activity into your daily life, and building a support network, fitness can become a lifelong habit that contributes to a healthier, more vibrant life.

11

Chapter 10: Personalized Programs and Next Steps

Creating Your Customized Plan

Creating your customized plan involves tailoring an exercise routine that meets your specific needs, goals, and limitations. It's about choosing the right mix of exercises that target different aspects of fitness such as strength, endurance, and flexibility. This customization is not a one-size-fits-all approach but rather an evolving strategy that adapts as you progress. The goal is to create a personalized plan that keeps you engaged, motivated, and progressing toward your fitness goals. This plan will evolve over time, allowing you to stay adaptable and continue enjoying the benefits of a healthy, active lifestyle.

Choosing the right exercises for your needs.

Choosing the right exercises for your needs is about matching the activities you select with your specific fitness goals, physical capabilities, and any health considerations you may have. It's about ensuring that each exercise you do contributes effectively to your overall fitness objectives.

First, consider your fitness goals. Are you looking to build muscle strength, improve cardiovascular endurance, enhance flexibility, or a combination of these? Different exercises target different aspects of fitness, so your choices should align with your primary objectives. For instance, if your goal is to build muscle strength, exercises such as weightlifting, resistance bands, and bodyweight exercises that challenge your muscles will be more suitable. If your goal is to improve cardiovascular health, exercises like walking, jogging, cycling, or swimming that get your heart pumping are key. If you're focused on flexibility, incorporating yoga, Pilates, or stretching routines will be beneficial.

Next, assess your current fitness level and any limitations you might have. This involves understanding your body's strengths and weaknesses and selecting exercises that are appropriate for your level of fitness. For beginners, starting with lighter weights, bodyweight exercises, or low-impact activities can help build confidence and reduce the risk of injury. For individuals with specific health conditions, such as arthritis, back pain, or joint issues, exercises that are gentle on the joints and don't cause discomfort should be prioritized. A physiotherapist or fitness professional can be particularly helpful in guiding these selections.

Consider the time you can commit to exercise and how frequently you can fit it into your schedule. Some people may prefer shorter, more intense workouts, while others might choose longer, moderate sessions. Your exercise choices should align with your lifestyle and be sustainable in the long term. For instance, if you have a busy schedule, quick, high-intensity interval training (HIIT) workouts might be more feasible than longer sessions. Similarly, if you enjoy social aspects of exercise, group classes or team sports could be a good fit.

Lastly, think about how the exercises will fit into your routine in terms of progression. As you get fitter, you'll want to continue challenging yourself by gradually increasing the intensity, resistance, or duration of your workouts. This could mean moving from bodyweight exercises to using weights, increasing repetitions, or changing exercises to target different muscle groups. The right exercises will not only help you achieve your immediate goals but also adapt as your fitness levels improve.

Balancing strength, endurance, and flexibility.

Balancing strength, endurance, and flexibility is about creating a well-rounded fitness routine that addresses all aspects of physical health. Each component—strength, endurance, and flexibility—plays a vital role in overall well-being and contributes to a balanced and sustainable fitness regimen.

Strength training focuses on building muscle mass and improving muscle strength. It involves exercises that challenge the muscles to contract against resistance, whether that's through weightlifting, resistance bands, bodyweight exercises, or even water resistance. Building strength not only helps improve posture and prevent injuries but also enhances daily activities such as lifting, carrying, and even climbing stairs. As you progress, it's important to include a variety of exercises that target different muscle groups, from the major muscle groups like legs, back, and chest to smaller muscle groups like arms, shoulders, and core. This diversity ensures balanced muscle development and prevents overuse injuries.

Endurance training, on the other hand, is about increasing the efficiency of the cardiovascular and respiratory systems, allowing you to sustain physical activity for longer periods without fatigue. This type of training improves stamina, which is crucial for daily activities and sports performance. It can be achieved through aerobic exercises such as walking, jogging, cycling, swimming, dancing, or even using cardio machines like treadmills and ellipticals. By incorporating endurance exercises into your routine, you strengthen your heart and lungs, which translates to improved overall health and the ability to engage in more strenuous physical activities as you age.

Flexibility is the ability of muscles and joints to move through their full range of motion without discomfort or pain. It's essential for maintaining a healthy, functional body and reducing the risk of injury. Stretching exercises, yoga, and Pilates are effective methods to improve flexibility. They help lengthen muscles, maintain joint health, and improve posture. A flexible body can move more efficiently, adapt to changes, and recover quicker from physical exertion.

Balancing these three components means integrating exercises that address all areas into your fitness plan. A well-rounded routine includes strength training to build muscle, endurance exercises to improve cardiovascular health, and flexibility exercises to enhance range of motion and prevent stiffness. This balanced approach ensures that you develop a complete fitness profile, allowing you to enjoy a higher quality of life, perform daily tasks more easily, and adapt to new physical challenges without overemphasizing one area at the expense of the others. Adjustments can be made based on individual goals, age, fitness level, and health considerations, but the key is to maintain a harmonious mix that supports overall physical health.

Modifying the program as you progress.

Modifying the program as you progress is an essential aspect of creating a sustainable fitness routine that evolves with your changing needs and capabilities. As you become more consistent with your exercise regimen and improve your fitness level, it's important to adapt the program to continue challenging yourself and ensuring ongoing progress. This flexibility allows for long-term success and helps prevent plateaus, burnout, or injury.

When you begin a fitness program, it's typically designed to introduce you to the basic exercises and routines needed to build a foundation. As you get stronger, more flexible, or your endurance improves, your body will require new challenges to keep progressing. This is where modifications come in. They might involve adjusting the intensity, volume, frequency, or type of exercises you perform. Here's how modifying the program works:

Adjusting Intensity:

Initially, you may start with low to moderate intensity exercises to ensure proper form and to minimize the risk of injury. As you progress, you can gradually increase the intensity—such as lifting heavier weights, adding more repetitions, or increasing the speed and resistance of cardio exercises. This can help stimulate muscle growth, improve cardiovascular fitness, and enhance overall strength and endurance.

Changing Exercise Selection:

As you gain more experience and your fitness level improves, you might need to introduce more advanced exercises or variations to continue your progress. For instance, if you started with basic squats, you might eventually incorporate variations like split squats or Bulgarian split squats to target different muscle groups more effectively. Similarly, if you began with basic walking, you might progress to jogging or interval training to enhance your cardiovascular capacity.

Adjusting Frequency and Duration:

Initially, you may begin with two to three sessions per week, gradually increasing to four or five as your body adapts. Modifying the program also means adjusting the duration of workouts. For example, if you started with 20-minute sessions, you might extend them to 30 or 45 minutes as you build stamina and capacity.

Tailoring to Specific Goals:

As you progress, your goals may change. Perhaps you initially wanted to improve general fitness, but now you have specific goals such as running a 5K, building upper body strength, or increasing flexibility. Modifying the program means selecting exercises and routines that align with these new objectives. For instance, if your goal is to run longer distances, you might include more endurance-focused workouts and recovery techniques. If you aim to improve strength, you may focus more on resistance training and modify the exercises to be heavier or more challenging.

Periodization:

Periodization is a method of organizing your workouts into cycles or phases over weeks or months to prevent overtraining and optimize performance. It involves varying the intensity, volume, and types of exercises across different periods. For example, you might go through a strength phase where you focus on building muscle mass, followed by an endurance phase that emphasizes cardiovascular fitness, and finally a maintenance phase that balances both aspects. This structured approach allows for steady progress and ensures that all fitness aspects are addressed throughout the year.

Monitoring Feedback:

As you progress, it's important to track your progress—through workouts, achievements, and self-assessment—to make informed adjustments. If you notice that certain exercises are becoming too easy, it's a sign that you need to modify the program to maintain a challenge. Conversely, if an exercise becomes too difficult and is causing discomfort or injury, you may need to scale back, modify the intensity, or substitute with a different exercise until your body adapts.

By continuously modifying the program based on your progress, you not only maximize your results but also keep the workouts engaging and prevent the risk of stagnation. This approach ensures that your fitness journey remains dynamic and aligned with your evolving fitness goals and lifestyle.

Integrating Fitness into Daily Life

Integrating fitness into daily life is about making physical activity a natural part of your routine, so it becomes sustainable over the long term. This approach helps maintain a healthy lifestyle without requiring a significant time investment. It's about finding creative ways to stay active and incorporating movement into everyday tasks.

Incorporating strength training into household chores.

Incorporating strength training into household chores involves turning daily tasks into opportunities to engage in physical activity that can strengthen muscles, improve endurance, and maintain overall fitness. This approach helps make fitness a more integral part of daily life without needing extra time or specialized equipment. It's about using your body weight and common household items as tools for resistance training, which can contribute to muscle maintenance and strength gains.

When you incorporate strength training into chores, you perform tasks with intentional effort to engage your muscles. For instance, lifting heavy grocery bags or pushing a vacuum cleaner can be done with a focus on controlled movements that challenge your muscles. Bending and lifting when gardening, cleaning windows, or moving furniture can be done in a way that strengthens the core, legs, and upper body. Squatting to pick up items, rather than bending over, not only protects your back but also works your quads, hamstrings, and glutes.

This approach can be adapted to any chore you're doing—whether it's doing laundry, loading and unloading the dishwasher, or even walking the dog. The key is to find opportunities to increase the effort required to complete these tasks, making them slightly more strenuous to enhance their fitness benefits. By integrating strength training into everyday chores, you can maintain muscle tone, improve cardiovascular health, and promote functional fitness, all while taking care of necessary tasks around the house. This method helps bridge the gap between traditional strength training exercises and real-life activities, making it easier to maintain a well-rounded fitness routine that fits seamlessly into your lifestyle.

Finding opportunities for movement throughout the day.

Finding opportunities for movement throughout the day involves creating habits that incorporate physical activity into your daily routine, regardless of whether you are at home, at work, or out running errands. It's about breaking up sedentary periods with short bursts of movement to keep your body active and your metabolism engaged. This approach helps combat the negative effects of prolonged sitting and ensures that you remain active even in busy or low-energy times.

Opportunities for movement can be as simple as taking a few minutes to stretch or do a few squats during TV breaks, taking the stairs instead of the elevator, or parking farther away from your destination to add an extra walk. If you work from home, setting a timer to remind yourself to stand up, walk around, or perform a quick workout during breaks can be highly effective. It's also about integrating physical activity into common tasks, such as walking while on the phone, using a standing desk if possible, or even doing light exercises like calf raises or seated marches while working at your desk.

In a broader sense, it can mean finding creative ways to incorporate movement into everyday activities—whether it's using a broom as a prop for balance exercises, engaging in light gardening, or taking a short walk after meals. The goal is to keep moving throughout the day, rather than having long periods of inactivity. This approach not only helps with physical health but also contributes to mental clarity, energy levels, and overall well-being. By weaving these small opportunities for movement into your daily life, you're more likely to maintain an active lifestyle that supports long-term health.

Staying active during travel or busy times.

Staying active during travel or busy times requires some planning and creativity to ensure that physical activity remains a priority, even when schedules are packed or routines are disrupted. This approach helps maintain fitness levels and keeps your body moving despite being on the go or dealing with tight deadlines.

During travel, whether it's for business or pleasure, finding ways to stay active can be integrated into the daily itinerary. This could mean planning a short morning run or walk around a new city, using hotel gyms or fitness centers, or finding nearby parks or trails to explore. Many airports now offer facilities for stretching or yoga, making it easier to sneak in some physical activity during layovers. You can also pack resistance bands or small fitness equipment that can be used in hotel rooms to perform a quick, effective workout.

For busy times when your schedule is packed with work, family obligations, or other commitments, staying active requires a commitment to integrate movement into those moments. This could mean opting for a walking meeting with a colleague, doing quick workouts at home between tasks, or finding opportunities to stretch and move during work breaks. Even small changes can make a difference—taking the stairs, standing up to do a few stretches during TV time, or walking around the block during lunch breaks.

The key is to remain adaptable and creative. Staying active during travel or busy times doesn't require an intense workout regimen but rather finding ways to move more frequently throughout the day. This might involve parking farther away, choosing to walk instead of drive, or even doing simple exercises like leg lifts or seated marches while working at a desk. The goal is to keep your body engaged and active, so you're not left feeling sluggish or stressed when busy periods subside.

Continuing Your Fitness Journey

Continuing your fitness journey requires a commitment to long-term health and wellbeing. Setting long-term fitness goals is an important first step. These goals can be anything from improving physical strength, enhancing cardiovascular health, increasing flexibility, or simply maintaining an active lifestyle as you age. Long-term goals provide a roadmap for your fitness journey and help you track progress over time. They should be specific, measurable, achievable, relevant, and time-bound to keep you motivated and on track.

Exploring group classes or senior fitness communities can be a great way to stay engaged and motivated. These settings offer structured workouts led by experienced instructors, which can provide a sense of camaraderie and encouragement. They also allow you to try new activities in a supportive environment, from gentle yoga and tai chi to strength training and aerobic exercises. Connecting with others who share similar fitness goals can help you stay inspired and accountable, and it can be an opportunity to make new friends and enjoy social interactions.

Staying inspired to age gracefully and actively involves embracing a mindset that values physical activity as a key component of a healthy lifestyle. It's about recognizing that fitness isn't just for the young but is a lifelong journey that can be enjoyed at any age. This might mean finding new forms of exercise that are enjoyable and sustainable, setting new personal records, or simply appreciating the benefits of physical activity for mental and emotional well-being. The journey is as much about the process as it is about the goals, and maintaining motivation can involve celebrating small achievements, setting new challenges, and continually seeking ways to improve and adapt your fitness routine.

12

CONCLUSION:

As we reach the conclusion of "Strength Training for Seniors Over 60: Adapted Programs for Older Adults with Limited Endurance," it's important to reflect on the journey we've taken together. Throughout this book, we've explored the fundamental principles of strength training tailored specifically for older adults. We began by understanding the importance of safety and assessing individual fitness levels, recognizing limitations, and consulting with a doctor before starting any new fitness program. We then delved into building a safe workout environment and developing a positive mindset, addressing fear and doubt, setting intentions, and celebrating small victories along the way.

We discussed the importance of proper equipment, including resistance bands, dumbbells, and other tools, and emphasized the need for correct posture and ergonomics to prevent injury. We covered the significance of frequency and duration in exercise, balancing rest and activity for recovery, and structuring a weekly fitness plan that can be integrated into daily life. We also explored intensity and progression, starting with low-intensity workouts, gradually increasing resistance and repetitions, and recognizing when to adjust routines as your strength improves.

Our focus shifted to specific muscle groups—upper body, core, lower body, and flexibility—highlighting exercises that enhance strength, balance, and coordination, as well as the role of functional movements in daily tasks.

CONCLUSION:

We discussed the benefits of resistance bands, dumbbells, and low-impact alternatives like chair-based training and pool exercises, ensuring that the workouts were accessible and suited to older adults with limited endurance.

The importance of flexibility and mobility was also underscored, with routines designed to prevent stiffness, improve range of motion, and promote relaxation and recovery. We talked about how gentle joint exercises, balance drills, and yoga-inspired moves can enhance overall wellbeing. We addressed common setbacks like injuries and health issues, reframing negative thoughts into motivation, and creating a support network for encouragement. We also discussed the need for consistency, setting a regular workout schedule, finding enjoyment in routines, and making fitness a lifelong habit.

This book aimed to provide a comprehensive guide to strength training for seniors, recognizing that every individual's journey is unique. Whether you're just starting out or have been active throughout your life, it's never too late to prioritize your health and fitness. The strategies and exercises shared here are adaptable to your individual needs and limitations, ensuring that you can achieve your goals safely and effectively.

Thank you for taking the time to read "Strength Training for Seniors Over 60." I hope you found the information helpful and inspiring as you embark on or continue your fitness journey. If you found value in this book, I would greatly appreciate it if you could take a moment to leave a review on Amazon. Your feedback helps others who are considering the same path to get the support they need. Best wishes on your journey to better health and a more active lifestyle!

13

QUIZ SECTION:

Here are 100 questions suitable for a quiz section based on the book *Strength Training for Seniors Over 60: Adapted Programs for Older Adults with Limited Endurance*:

1. What is the first step you should take before starting a new fitness program?
2. Why is it important to consult with a doctor before starting a fitness program?
3. What role does setting a positive mindset play in starting a fitness journey?
4. Which equipment is commonly recommended for beginners in strength training?
5. Why is proper posture crucial when performing exercises?
6. How often should seniors exercise according to the book?
7. What is the importance of balancing rest and activity?
8. What is a key aspect of structuring a weekly fitness plan?
9. Why is it important to start with low-intensity workouts?
10. What does gradually increasing resistance help with?
11. What should you do when you recognize your routine is not challenging enough?
12. How do resistance bands enhance muscle engagement?

13. Why is flexibility important in a senior's fitness routine?
14. What kind of stretches are recommended before a workout?
15. What are dynamic stretches used for?
16. What is the benefit of static stretches after a workout?
17. How do yoga-inspired moves contribute to flexibility?
18. What are gentle joint exercises used for?
19. Why are balance drills important for seniors?
20. What functional movements are recommended for everyday tasks?
21. What should you do if you experience fatigue?
22. How does endurance contribute to overall fitness?
23. Why is it important to balance strength training with cardio exercises?
24. What type of chair exercises are beneficial for leg strength?
25. How do heel lifts help with ankle stability?
26. What is the purpose of weighted step-ups?
27. What kind of dumbbells should seniors use for safety?
28. Why are wrist curls important for forearm endurance?
29. What is the benefit of seated rows for seniors?
30. How can weighted lunges benefit leg strength?
31. What is the importance of using light dumbbells for heel lifts?
32. How do dynamic stretches prepare seniors for exercise?
33. What is the role of yoga-inspired moves in improving balance?
34. Why should seniors incorporate pool exercises into their routine?
35. What is the benefit of slow, controlled movements in workouts?
36. What should you do when managing injuries?
37. How can reframing negative thoughts improve motivation?
38. Why is a support network important for encouragement?
39. How do rest days benefit seniors?
40. What is active recovery, and how can it be achieved?
41. Why is monitoring progress important in fitness?
42. What are the benefits of journaling workouts and milestones?
43. How can you celebrate small wins during your fitness journey?
44. What should you do when setting long-term fitness goals?
45. What is the benefit of exploring group classes or senior fitness commu-

nities?

46. How does staying inspired help in aging gracefully?
47. Why is finding enjoyment important in a fitness routine?
48. How can strength training be incorporated into household chores?
49. What are the benefits of finding movement opportunities throughout the day?
50. How can seniors stay active during travel or busy times?
51. What should be considered when choosing exercises for your needs?
52. Why is balancing strength, endurance, and flexibility crucial in a fitness plan?
53. How can you modify a fitness program as you progress?
54. What are some examples of chair-based strength training exercises?
55. How do pool exercises help with joint relief?
56. What does it mean to perform slow, controlled movements in exercise?
57. How can you identify fatigue and modify intensity?
58. Why is it important to understand the role of endurance in fitness?
59. What should you balance strength with in terms of cardio for overall health?
60. What are some examples of chair squats?
61. How can calf raises improve ankle stability?
62. What is the purpose of step-ups in fitness routines?
63. How do dumbbell chest presses contribute to upper strength?
64. What are lateral raises used for in a senior's fitness routine?
65. Why are wrist curls important for forearm endurance?
66. What benefits do weighted lunges provide?
67. How do heel lifts with light dumbbells improve leg strength?
68. What is the benefit of weighted step-ups for balance?
69. How do dynamic stretches benefit a pre-workout routine?
70. Why are static stretches important for post-workout cool-downs?
71. What role do yoga-inspired moves play in improving flexibility?
72. How can gentle joint exercises reduce stiffness?
73. Why are balance drills crucial for preventing falls?
74. How do functional movements improve ease of daily tasks?

75. What should you do if you experience an injury or health issue?
76. How can negative thoughts be reframed into motivation?
77. What role does a support network play in encouragement?
78. Why are rest days important for seniors?
79. What are some examples of active recovery techniques?
80. How should you monitor progress in a fitness program?
81. What are some milestones to track in fitness journaling?
82. How do you celebrate small wins during your journey?
83. Why should you adjust goals as you improve?
84. How can you maintain a regular workout schedule?
85. What steps can you take to find enjoyment in your fitness routine?
86. Why is it important to keep fitness a lifelong habit?
87. How can strength training be incorporated into daily chores?
88. What opportunities exist for movement throughout the day?
89. How can seniors stay active during travel?
90. What should be considered when setting long-term fitness goals?
91. Why are group classes beneficial for seniors?
92. How can you stay inspired to age gracefully and actively?
93. How do you choose the right exercises for your needs?
94. What does balancing strength, endurance, and flexibility involve?
95. How should you modify a fitness program as you progress?
96. What role does finding enjoyment play in sticking to a fitness routine?
97. How can strength training be seamlessly integrated into household chores?
98. What is a key benefit of finding movement opportunities throughout the day?
99. How can seniors stay active during travel or busy times?
100. Why is setting long-term fitness goals important for continued motivation?

www.ingramcontent.com/pod-product-compliance
Lightning Source LLC
Chambersburg PA
CBHW051614250726

48653CB00004BA/1504